Knowing is Key

Herbs and Roots: Unlocking Nature's Power

By: Chickamooka Love

"WITHIN EVERY HERB LIES THE WISDOM OF NATURE; A QUIET POWER TO SOOTHE, NOURISH, AND RESTORE BALANCE TO THE BODY AND SOUL."

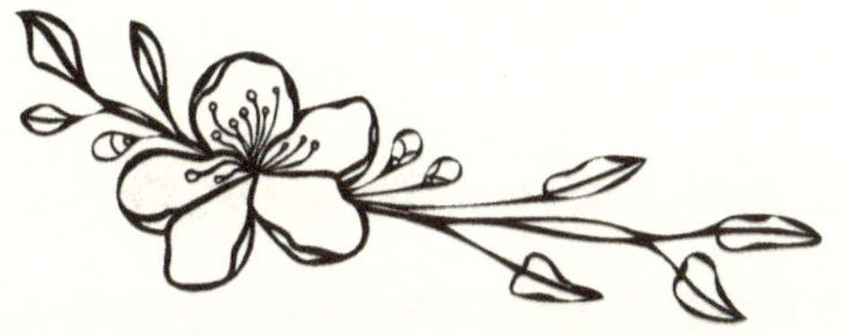

Herbs are highly versatile and can be used in many forms such as teas, tinctures, powders, essential oils, and more depending on the desired effect. By understanding their properties, you can tap into the natural wisdom of the herbs power.

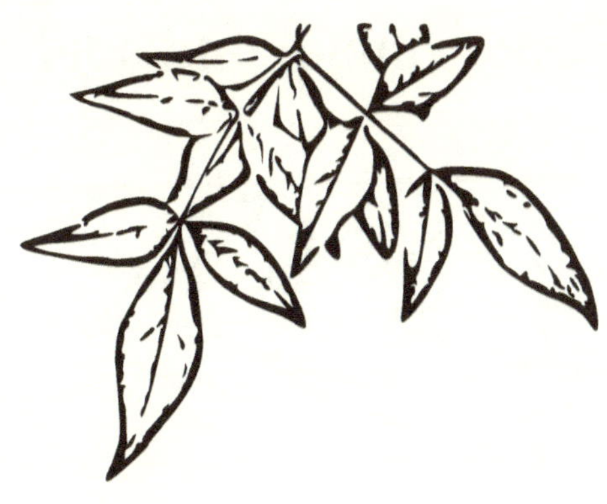

Herbs are a rich and diverse category of plants used across time and cultures for their healing, culinary, and spiritual properties. They contain bioactive compounds that influence bodily functions and offer a natural, holistic approach to health. Whether in traditional remedies, modern medicine, or everyday cooking, herbs continue to play a central role in human life, offering their quiet power to nourish, protect, and restore balance to the body, mind, and soul.

Types of Herbs

Culinary Herbs: Used primarily for flavoring and enhancing food. Examples include basil, oregano, thyme, and cilantro. Culinary herbs usually have mild aromatic properties that elevate the taste of dishes.

Medicinal Herbs: Used for healing purposes, either in traditional medicine or modern herbal therapy. Examples include echinacea, ginseng, and turmeric. These herbs contain active compounds that affect bodily functions and can treat or prevent various health conditions.

Aromatic Herbs: Valued for their scent and are used in perfumes, incense, and essential oils. Lavender, rosemary, and mint are examples of aromatic herbs that are used in both medicinal and cosmetic applications.

Spiritual Herbs: Often used in rituals, ceremonies, or as offerings. Examples include sage for smudging, frankincense, and sandalwood, which are burned for spiritual cleansing and creating sacred spaces.

Properties of Herbs

Alkaloids: Potent compounds that can have medicinal or toxic effects, depending on the dosage. Examples include the alkaloid caffeine in tea and coffee, and berberine in goldenseal, which has antimicrobial properties.

Flavonoids: Antioxidants that protect the body from free radicals, reducing oxidative stress and inflammation. They are often responsible for the bright colors in fruits and herbs.

Terpenes: Aromatic compounds found in essential oils that can have medicinal properties, such as anti-inflammatory, antiviral, or antimicrobial effects. They are found in herbs like lavender, rosemary, and eucalyptus.

Saponins: Compounds that have cleansing and immune-boosting properties, found in plants like licorice and yucca.

Tannins: Astringent compounds that can be used to heal wounds and improve digestive health. Tannins are present in herbs like witch hazel and oak bark.

Herbs in History and Culture

Ancient Civilizations: Herbs have been used for thousands of years in traditional healing practices across many ancient civilizations:

The Egyptians used herbs like garlic and coriander in both medicine and food. They also buried herbs with their dead as part of the mummification process.

The Chinese developed a highly sophisticated herbal medicine system that still exists today. The book Shennong Bencao Jing is one of the earliest pharmacopoeias, listing hundreds of herbs and their uses.

The Greeks and Romans used herbs in their daily lives for medicine, food, and ritual. Hippocrates, known as the "Father of Medicine," often recommended herbs like sage and thyme for healing.

Ayurveda: In India, the ancient system of Ayurveda uses herbs to maintain balance between the body, mind, and spirit. Herbs like turmeric, ashwagandha, and Tulsi are essential to this tradition.

Native American Practices: Indigenous peoples of the Americas used a variety of herbs like sage, tobacco, and echinacea for medicinal, spiritual, and ceremonial purposes.

Modern Uses of Herbs

Alternative Medicine: Many people now use herbs as part of alternative medicine or holistic health practices. Herbs like echinacea are used to boost the immune system, while chamomile and valerian are used for calming and aiding sleep.

Cosmetic and Aromatherapy: Essential oils extracted from herbs are used for skin care, relaxation, and overall wellness. Lavender oil, for example, is used for its soothing properties in aromatherapy.

Food and Beverages: Herbs play a major role in the culinary world, from flavoring dishes to creating herbal teas that promote health. Green tea, for instance, is rich in antioxidants and is valued for its detoxifying properties.

How Herbs Work in the Body

Modulating the immune system: Some herbs, such as astragalus and echinacea, help boost the body's immune response, aiding in the prevention of infections and illnesses.

Balancing hormones: Herbs like maca root and vitex are often used to support hormonal balance, especially in women's health for issues like PMS or menopause.

Supporting digestion: Bitter herbs like dandelion and gentian stimulate digestive enzymes and bile production, improving digestion and nutrient absorption.

Anti-inflammatory action: Many herbs, like turmeric and ginger, contain compounds that reduce inflammation in the body, helping with conditions like arthritis or inflammatory bowel disease.

Calming the nervous system: Herbs like valerian root and passionflower are used for their sedative properties, helping to relieve anxiety and insomnia.

Perennial Herb

A perennial herb is a type of plant that lives for more than two years and produces new growth season after season. Unlike annual herbs, which complete their life cycle in one growing season, or biennial herbs, which live for two years, perennial herbs regrow every spring from the same root system, although they may die back in winter in colder climates.

Longevity: Perennial herbs can live and produce for several years, making them a long-lasting addition to gardens.

Growth Cycle: These herbs typically go through periods of active growth (spring and summer), dormancy (fall and winter), and regrowth the following season.

Hardiness: Many perennial herbs are hardy and can survive through harsh weather conditions, often dying back to the roots in winter but reemerging in spring.

Low Maintenance: Once established, perennial herbs usually require less care than annuals, as they don't need to be replanted every year.

Examples of Perennial Herbs

Mint (Mentha spp.): Known for its invasive growth, mint is a vigorous perennial herb that returns year after year.

Thyme (Thymus vulgaris): A low-growing herb used in cooking, thyme is a hardy perennial that thrives in sunny spots.

Lavender (Lavandula spp.): A fragrant herb used in both culinary and medicinal preparations, lavender is a popular perennial known for its beautiful purple flowers.

Sage (Salvia officinalis): This woody perennial is often used in cooking and for medicinal purposes. Sage can live for many years with proper care.

Oregano (Origanum vulgare): Another culinary staple, oregano is a hardy perennial often used in Mediterranean cooking.

Advantages of Perennial Herbs:

Cost-effective: Since they don't need to be replanted every year, perennial herbs save time and money.

Sustainability: Perennials tend to improve soil structure and contribute to healthier ecosystems.

Continuous Harvest: Once established, perennial herbs provide a consistent and reliable harvest year after year, often with minimal care.

Perennial herbs are an excellent choice for gardeners looking for low-maintenance, sustainable plants that offer repeated harvests of fresh herbs throughout the growing seasons.

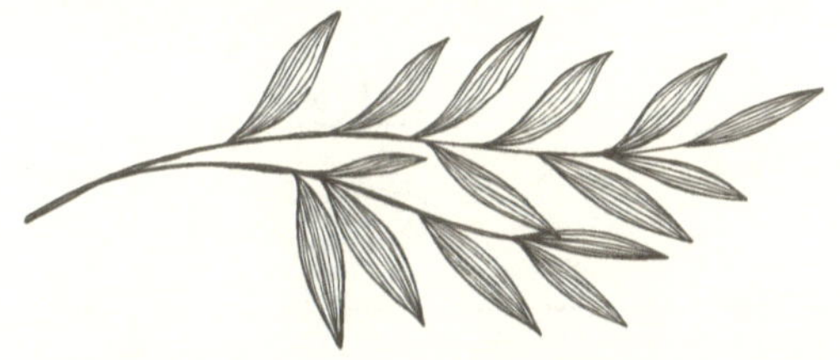

Spiritual and Symbolic Meanings

Herbs are often tied to spiritual traditions, where they are seen as sacred gifts of the Earth. For example:

Sage: Used in Native American traditions for smudging and clearing negative energy.

Frankincense and Myrrh: Common in the Middle Eastern rituals for purification.

Basil: Known as the "holy herb" in many cultures and used in rituals to bring protection and harmony.

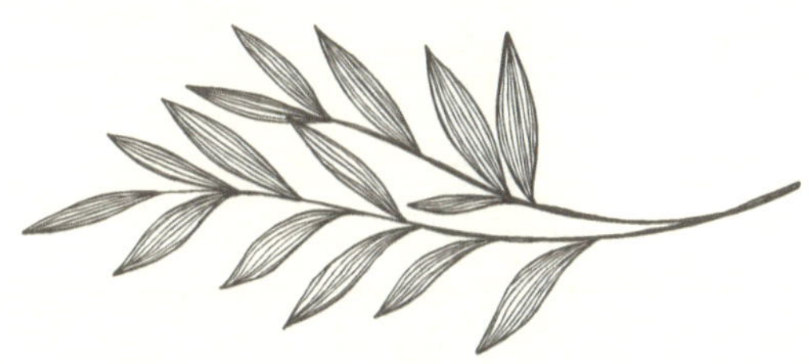

Knowing

Date:

Knowing Date: ____________

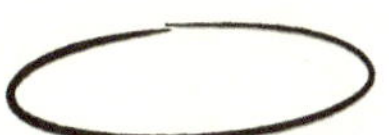

Knowing Date: ______________

Knowing Date: ____________

Knowing

Date: ____________

Knowing Date: ____________

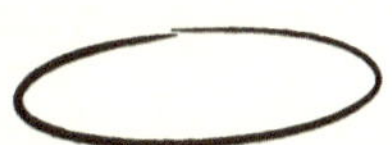

Dandelion (Taraxacum officinale)

Common Names:

Dandelion, Lion's Tooth, Blowball, Cankerwort, Fairy Clock

Botanical Name:

Taraxacum officinale

Family: Asteraceae (Daisy family)

Type: Perennial herb

Origin: Native to Europe and Asia, dandelion now grows worldwide and is often considered a weed. However, its leaves, flowers, and roots have been prized in herbal medicine and traditional foods for centuries.

Plant Description

Dandelions are hardy, perennial herbs with bright yellow flowers and jagged, toothed leaves. The entire plant is edible and has a wide range of medicinal uses. Dandelions are easily recognized by their sunny flowers and round, white seed heads that spread seeds when blown by the wind.

Key Features

Height: Dandelions grow to a height of about 4–18 inches (10–45 cm).

Leaves: The leaves are jagged and toothed, growing directly from the base in a rosette. They are deep green and can be used as salad greens when young.

Flowers: Bright yellow flowers appear in early spring and bloom throughout the season. They are composite flowers, meaning each "flower" is a collection of many small florets.

Roots: Dandelion has a long, thick taproot that grows deep into the soil. This root is commonly used in herbal preparations.

Medicinal Properties

Dandelion is known for its diuretic, detoxifying, digestive, anti-inflammatory, and nutritive properties. Each part of the plant has unique benefits, making it a versatile and widely used herb in herbal medicine.

Liver Health and Detoxification: Dandelion is often used as a liver tonic, as it is believed to stimulate bile production and support healthy liver function. This makes it helpful in cleansing the body, promoting detoxification, and potentially alleviating skin conditions linked to poor liver function.

Digestive Health: Dandelion root acts as a mild digestive bitter. It stimulates appetite, increases saliva and digestive enzyme production, and can alleviate symptoms of bloating, gas, and sluggish digestion. Dandelion leaves, rich in potassium, also support kidney function by acting as a gentle diuretic.

Diuretic: Dandelion leaves have a natural diuretic effect, which increases urine production without causing potassium depletion, a common side effect of synthetic diuretics. This property makes it useful for reducing water retention, promoting kidney health, and supporting the body's natural detoxification processes.

Anti-Inflammatory and Antioxidant: Dandelion contains antioxidant compounds, including polyphenols and beta-carotene, which help to combat inflammation and oxidative stress in the body. These properties are beneficial for protecting cells from damage and reducing chronic inflammation.

Nutritive Properties: Dandelion is a rich source of vitamins A, C, K, and some B vitamins, as well as minerals like iron, calcium, magnesium, and potassium. It is particularly valued as a nutrient-dense food and a nourishing herb for overall vitality.

Interesting Facts

Common Weed and Medicine: Although often considered a common garden weed, dandelion's medicinal properties have earned it a respected place in herbal medicine for thousands of years.

Culinary Uses

Dandelion is edible from root to flower and has a long history as a nutritious wild green. The young leaves can be added to salads, and the roots can be roasted or sautéed. Flowers can be used to make dandelion wine or added to salads for a pop of color and mild flavor.

Traditional and Modern Uses

Internal Uses

Tea or Infusion: Dandelion root or leaf tea is one of the most common ways to use dandelion. Root tea is generally used for liver and digestive support, while leaf tea serves as a gentle diuretic.
Tincture: Dandelion tinctures, made from roots, leaves, or a combination, offer a concentrated form of the herb. These tinctures are often used to support liver function and digestion.
Capsules or Powder: Dandelion is available in capsule or powdered form for convenience. These are especially popular for people who prefer not to taste the bitterness of the plant but want the benefits for liver health and detox.
Dandelion Coffee: Roasted dandelion root can be brewed as a caffeine-free coffee substitute. This "dandelion coffee" has a rich, slightly bitter flavor and is valued for supporting liver function and digestion.

External Uses

Poultice or Salve: Dandelion flowers can be infused into oil to make a healing salve for sore muscles, minor wounds, or dry skin. The flowers are mildly anti-inflammatory and soothing when applied topically.
Skin Tonic: Dandelion leaf infusions can be used as a skin toner or added to baths. Dandelion is considered beneficial for reducing skin inflammation and may help with acne and other skin conditions related to toxicity.

How to Harvest

Leaves: Young, tender leaves are best harvested in the spring before the plant flowers, as they become more bitter with age.

Flowers: Dandelion flowers should be picked in the morning when fully open, as they tend to close up later in the day. They are best used fresh for making infusions or dandelion oil.

Roots: The roots are ideally harvested in the fall when the plant stores more nutrients in the root. They can be dug up, cleaned, dried, or roasted for use in teas or other preparations.

Precautions

Allergic Reactions: Some individuals may be allergic to dandelion, especially those with allergies to plants in the Asteraceae family. Discontinue use if any allergic reactions occur.

Medication Interactions: Due to its diuretic effect, dandelion may interfere with certain medications, especially diuretics, blood thinners, and medications for blood pressure. Consult a healthcare provider if taking any prescription medications.

Bile Duct Obstruction: Dandelion should be avoided by people with blocked bile ducts, as it stimulates bile production, which could exacerbate the condition.

Energetics

In traditional herbalism, dandelion is considered cooling and drying. Its bitter and astringent qualities make it valuable for clearing heat and reducing stagnation in the liver and digestive system. It's often used to address conditions related to "dampness" and "heat" in the body, such as sluggish digestion, bloating, and skin issues.

Conclusion

Dandelion is a truly versatile herb, renowned for its diuretic, detoxifying, and digestive-supporting properties. Each part of the plant offers unique benefits, from the nutrient-rich leaves to the detoxifying roots. Widely used to support liver function and healthy digestion, dandelion is considered a cleansing and restorative herb. With its high nutrient content and gentle yet effective properties, dandelion serves as both a food and a medicinal herb, often used as a tea, tincture, or topical application.

Elderberry (Sambucus nigra)

Common Names:

Elderberry, European Elder, Black Elder

Botanical Name:

Sambucus nigra

Family: Adoxaceae (Moschatel family)

Type: Perennial shrub

Origin: Native to Europe, North America, and parts of Asia. Elderberry has a long tradition in herbal medicine, especially in Europe and North America, where it has been used by indigenous tribes and in folk remedies for centuries.

Plant Description

Elderberry is a deciduous shrub or small tree that thrives in moist, well-drained soils and can often be found growing wild along riverbanks, roadsides, and forest edges. It is renowned for its dark purple berries and fragrant, creamy white flowers, both of which are used in herbal medicine.

Key Features

Height: Elderberry shrubs typically grow between 6 to 12 feet (1.8 to 3.6 meters) tall, though they can reach up to 20 feet (6 meters) in ideal conditions.

Leaves: The leaves are pinnate, meaning they are divided into several leaflets arranged along a central stem. They are serrated, dark green, and grow in pairs.

Flowers: Elderberry produces clusters of small, white to pale yellow flowers in early summer. The flowers have a pleasant fragrance and are also used medicinally.

Fruits: Elderberries are small, round, and dark purple to black when ripe, typically growing in large clusters. The berries ripen in late summer to early fall and are known for their high antioxidant content and immune-supporting properties.

Medicinal Properties

Elderberry is rich in antioxidants, vitamin C, flavonoids, and anthocyanins, all of which contribute to its immune-boosting effects. It is also recognized for its antiviral and anti-inflammatory properties, making it a valuable herb for treating colds, flu, and other respiratory infections.

Immune Support and Cold Relief: Elderberry is widely used to support the immune system, particularly in fighting off cold and flu viruses. The berries contain compounds that inhibit the attachment and replication of viruses, making them effective for shortening the duration and severity of colds and flu. Elderberry syrup, in particular, is popular as a preventive and treatment remedy during cold and flu season.

Antioxidant Protection: Elderberries are packed with antioxidants, especially anthocyanins, which give the berries their deep purple color. These antioxidants help neutralize free radicals, reducing oxidative stress in the body and protecting cells from damage. This, in turn, supports overall health and may help prevent chronic diseases.

Anti-Inflammatory Effects: Elderberry has natural anti-inflammatory properties, which can help reduce swelling and pain associated with colds, sinus infections, and inflammation in the respiratory tract. This is beneficial for conditions like sinusitis, where reducing inflammation can help relieve congestion and improve breathing.

Respiratory Health: Elderberry is often used to alleviate symptoms of respiratory conditions, such as bronchitis and sinus congestion. It helps to clear mucus from the respiratory tract and may soothe sore throats. Elderberry tea or syrup is commonly taken to relieve coughs and congestion.

Digestive Health: Elderberry has mild laxative properties, which can help relieve constipation and promote regular bowel movements. The berries contain dietary fiber that supports digestive health and aids in detoxifying the body.

Skin Health: Elderberry's antioxidant and anti-inflammatory properties can also benefit the skin. Elderberry extracts are used in skincare products to combat signs of aging, such as wrinkles and fine lines, and to promote a clear, glowing complexion. The flavonoids in elderberries help protect the skin from UV damage and environmental stressors.

Culinary Uses

While elderberries are highly nutritious, they must be cooked before consumption, as raw berries (and other parts of the plant, like leaves and stems) contain compounds that can cause nausea and digestive upset. Cooked elderberries can be used in syrups, jams, jellies, pies, and sauces. Elderflower, the plant's blossom, is also used in culinary recipes for teas, cordials, and desserts, adding a floral and lightly sweet flavor.

Traditional and Modern Uses

Internal Uses

Syrup: Elderberry syrup is one of the most common ways to consume elderberries. It's typically made by simmering elderberries with water and honey (or another sweetener) to create a thick, sweet syrup. Elderberry syrup is known for its immune-boosting effects and is taken regularly during cold and flu season for prevention and treatment.
Tea or Infusion: Elderberry tea is made by steeping dried berries or flowers in hot water. It is often consumed for its immune-boosting, antioxidant, and anti-inflammatory properties, particularly to relieve symptoms of colds, flu, and respiratory congestion.
Tincture: Elderberry tincture provides a concentrated form of the herb, which is useful for quick and easy immune support. It's taken in small, measured doses, often diluted in water.
Gummies: Elderberry gummies have become popular as a palatable, convenient way for both adults and children to consume elderberry for daily immune support.

External Uses

Skin Care: Elderberry extracts are used in skincare products for their anti-aging and anti-inflammatory effects. The berries' high antioxidant content helps protect the skin from free radicals, while their anti-inflammatory properties soothe irritation. Elderberry-infused lotions, creams, and serums are popular for promoting a healthy complexion.
Poultices: Elderberry leaves were traditionally used in poultices to treat wounds, bruises, and skin infections. The leaves contain mild antibacterial properties and were applied to help reduce swelling and promote healing.

How to Harvest

Berries: Elderberries are harvested in late summer to early fall when they are fully ripe and dark purple or black in color. The berries are typically cut in clusters and then gently removed from the stems, as the stems are not edible and contain toxic compounds. After harvesting, the berries are cooked or dried for later use.

Flowers: Elderflowers are harvested in early summer, just as the buds fully open. The flowers are used fresh or dried for teas, tinctures, and culinary recipes.

Precautions

Toxicity: Raw elderberries, as well as the leaves, stems, and roots, contain cyanogenic glycosides, which can release cyanide when ingested. These compounds are rendered harmless through cooking, so elderberries should always be cooked before consumption.

Allergic Reactions: Some individuals may be allergic to elderberry, especially if they are sensitive to other plants in the Adoxaceae family. Skin reactions or digestive discomfort may occur in rare cases.

Pregnancy and Nursing: Pregnant and nursing women should consult with a healthcare provider before using elderberry, as its safety in these groups is not fully established.

Energetics

In traditional herbal medicine, elderberry is considered cooling and drying. It is beneficial for conditions associated with excess heat, such as fever, inflammation, and viral infections. Elderberry is used to dispel toxins, clear heat, and promote a balanced immune response.

Interesting Facts

Modern Research: Recent studies have confirmed that elderberry can shorten the duration of cold and flu symptoms. Elderberry extract has been shown to prevent viral replication, boost cytokine production, and reduce the severity of symptoms in patients with influenza.

Conclusion

Elderberry is a versatile herb that has been valued for centuries for its immune-boosting and antiviral properties. As a powerful remedy for colds, flu, and other respiratory ailments, elderberry provides natural relief and support for the body's defenses. Its antioxidant, anti-inflammatory, and skin-nourishing properties also make it an excellent choice for overall wellness, and its versatility allows it to be used in a variety of ways, from syrups and teas to skincare. Elderberry's popularity as an immune-supportive herb endures, making it a staple in both traditional and modern herbal medicine.

Mullein (Verbascum Thapsus)

Common Names:

Mullein, Common Mullein, Great Mullein, Velvet Plant, Candlewick Plant

Botanical Name:

Verbascum Thapsus

Family: Scrophulariaceae (Figwort family)

Type: Biennial herb

Origin: Native to Europe, Asia, and North Africa; naturalized in North America. Mullein has been used in herbal medicine for centuries, primarily for respiratory health, and was valued by ancient Greek and Roman herbalists for its soothing properties.

Plant Description

Mullein is a distinctive and tall herb with a woolly appearance, especially popular for its tall, spike-like inflorescence and large, soft leaves. This hardy plant thrives in poor, dry soils and often grows along roadsides, in fields, and in disturbed areas.

Key Features

Height: Mullein can grow between 2 to 7 feet (0.6 to 2.1 meters) tall. In its first year, it forms a basal rosette of leaves, and in the second year, it sends up a tall flowering spike.

Leaves: The large, woolly leaves are soft and fuzzy, giving them a velvety feel. They form a basal rosette in the first year and grow alternately along the stem in the second year.

Flowers: Mullein produces small, pale yellow flowers on a tall, dense spike. The flowers bloom in succession from the bottom to the top of the spike during summer and have a mild, sweet fragrance.

Seeds: The tiny, dark seeds are produced in abundance and can remain viable in soil for decades, contributing to mullein's ability to spread easily.

Medicinal Properties

Mullein is renowned for its demulcent (soothing), expectorant, and anti-inflammatory properties, which make it especially useful for respiratory health. It is also known for its antiviral and antimicrobial effects.

Respiratory Health: Mullein is highly regarded as a remedy for respiratory ailments, including coughs, bronchitis, asthma, and congestion. It acts as a gentle expectorant, helping to loosen and expel mucus from the lungs, making it easier to breathe. Its soothing, anti-inflammatory effects help calm irritated airways and reduce inflammation in the respiratory tract.

Antiviral and Antibacterial: Mullein contains compounds that have shown antiviral and antibacterial activity, making it useful for infections in the respiratory system, like colds and flu. This antimicrobial property also helps prevent secondary infections that can sometimes follow viral respiratory illnesses.

Anti-Inflammatory and Pain Relief: Mullein's anti-inflammatory properties make it beneficial for reducing inflammation in the respiratory tract, easing pain in sore throats, and relieving aches associated with infections. Some traditional uses even extend to joint pain and muscle aches.

Ear Health: Mullein flower oil is commonly used as a remedy for ear infections and earaches, particularly in children. The oil has soothing, antibacterial, and analgesic properties that can relieve pain and reduce inflammation in the ear canal.

Skin Health: Mullein has mild antibacterial and soothing properties that make it effective in treating minor skin wounds, cuts, burns, and rashes. It can also be applied as a poultice for skin infections or to relieve pain and inflammation from insect bites and stings

Interesting Facts

Historical Use as Lamp Wicks: In ancient times, the dried stalks of mullein were dipped in tallow or wax and used as torches or "candlewicks," giving mullein its nickname "Candlewick Plant."

Traditional Lung Remedy: Mullein has been used for respiratory ailments since ancient times. The Greek physician Dioscorides recommended mullein for lung conditions over 2,000 years ago, and it remains a go-to herb for lung health today.

Folklore: In traditional folklore, mullein was sometimes called "Hag's Taper" and was believed to ward off evil spirits. It was often planted near doorways and was thought to provide protection.

Traditional and Modern Uses

Internal Uses

Tea or Infusion: Mullein tea, made from the dried leaves or flowers, is one of the most popular ways to use mullein. It is a gentle remedy for coughs, sore throats, and respiratory congestion. Mullein tea is usually strained to remove the tiny leaf hairs, which can be irritating if ingested.
Tincture: Mullein tinctures are made from the leaves or flowers and offer a concentrated form of the herb. Tinctures are commonly used for respiratory support, especially for chronic respiratory issues like asthma or bronchitis.
Syrup: Mullein syrup, often combined with honey, is another effective remedy for soothing sore throats and coughs. The syrup is especially useful during the cold and flu season for its mucilage, which coats and soothes irritated respiratory tissues.

External Uses

Ear Oil: Mullein flower oil is a well-known remedy for earaches and ear infections. It's often combined with garlic oil for enhanced antimicrobial effects and is applied in small amounts directly into the ear for relief.
Poultices and Compresses: Mullein leaves or flowers can be made into a poultice or compress to treat skin issues, including cuts, wounds, or insect bites. The leaves' anti-inflammatory and antibacterial properties make mullein beneficial for soothing and promoting healing.
Steam Inhalation: Mullein leaves are sometimes used in steam inhalation to relieve congestion and open up airways. Adding mullein leaves to a bowl of hot water and inhaling the steam can be helpful for colds, coughs, and sinus congestion.

How to Harvest

Leaves: Mullein leaves are best harvested in the first year when they are large and robust, but can also be gathered in the early part of the second year before the plant flowers. The leaves are typically dried and stored for teas and tinctures.

Flowers: Mullein flowers are harvested in the second year during blooming, usually from late spring to summer. The flowers are picked individually and are often used fresh in oil infusions or dried for later use in teas or tinctures.

Precautions

Straining Tea: Mullein leaves contain tiny hairs that can irritate the throat and digestive system if ingested. It is essential to strain mullein tea thoroughly through a fine mesh or cheesecloth before drinking.

Potential Skin Sensitivity: Some people may experience skin irritation when handling or using mullein leaves due to the fine hairs. Gloves can be worn during harvesting to prevent irritation.

Allergic Reactions: Although rare, some individuals may be sensitive or allergic to mullein. Anyone with known allergies to other members of the figwort family should use mullein cautiously.

Energetics

In traditional herbal medicine, mullein is considered cooling and drying. It is especially beneficial for conditions involving excess moisture, such as mucus congestion in the lungs. Mullein is used to clear phlegm, calm irritation, and restore balance in the respiratory tract.

Conclusion

Mullein is a time-honored herb, especially valued for its role in supporting respiratory health. From easing coughs and congestion to soothing inflammation in the lungs and throat, mullein provides natural relief for a variety of respiratory issues. Its versatility extends to ear health, skin care, and even minor pain relief, making it a well-rounded herb with a place in both traditional and modern herbal practices. With its gentle, soothing properties, mullein continues to be a valuable remedy for those seeking natural support for respiratory health and beyond.

Burdock (Arctium lappa)

Common Names:

Burdock, Gobo, Beggar's Buttons, Great Burdock

Botanical Name:

Arctium lappa

Family: Asteraceae (Daisy family)

Type: Biennial herb

Origin: Native to Europe and Northern Asia, burdock has naturalized throughout North America. It's valued as a traditional medicinal herb and is also widely used as a food in Japan and parts of Asia.

Plant Description

Burdock is a large biennial herb that can grow up to 6 feet tall, with broad, heart-shaped leaves and purple, thistle-like flowers. Known for its sticky seed heads or "burs," which cling to clothes and animal fur, burdock is primarily valued for its long, fibrous roots, used in herbal medicine and as a nutritious food.

Key Features

Height: Burdock can grow between 3–6 feet (1–2 meters) tall.

Leaves: The large, heart-shaped leaves are dark green and have a slightly fuzzy underside. They grow in a rosette at the base in the plant's first year, then produce a tall stalk in the second year.

Flowers: Burdock's flowers are purple and resemble thistles. They bloom in clusters at the tops of the stems and form prickly burs that aid seed dispersal.

Roots: The roots are long, thick, and brown, sometimes reaching 2–3 feet deep. They have a mild, earthy flavor when cooked and are the primary part used in herbal medicine.

Medicinal Properties

Burdock is known for its detoxifying, diuretic, anti-inflammatory, antioxidant, and blood-purifying properties. It is commonly used to support skin health, liver function, and detoxification.

Liver and Detox Support: Burdock root is valued as a liver tonic that promotes bile production and supports liver function, making it popular in detox formulas. By aiding the liver in filtering and processing toxins, burdock is believed to support overall body cleansing.

Blood Purifier: Burdock is traditionally used as a "blood purifier" in herbal medicine, which refers to its ability to remove toxins from the blood and promote better circulation. This makes it particularly helpful for conditions like acne, eczema, and other inflammatory skin issues that may be linked to internal imbalances.

Diuretic: Burdock root has mild diuretic properties, which help the body release excess water and toxins through the urine. This effect supports kidney function and overall fluid balance in the body, often helping to relieve mild edema.

Skin Health: Burdock root is widely known for its benefits to the skin. Due to its blood-cleansing and anti-inflammatory properties, it's often used to address skin issues like acne, eczema, and psoriasis. Its cooling nature makes it suitable for treating skin conditions associated with heat or inflammation.

Antioxidant: Burdock is rich in antioxidants, including quercetin, luteolin, and phenolic acids. These compounds protect cells from oxidative damage and help reduce inflammation in the body, offering overall health benefits and potentially slowing the aging process.

Interesting Facts

Inspiration for Velcro: Burdock burs were the inspiration for Velcro. Swiss engineer George de Mestral studied the structure of burdock seed heads and created the now-famous fastening system in the 1940s.

Traditional Use by Indigenous Peoples: Native American tribes and European herbalists have used burdock for centuries as a detoxifying tonic and for various skin issues. It was often prepared as a root tea or applied topically as a poultice.

Traditional and Modern Uses

Internal Uses

Tea or Decoction: Burdock root is commonly prepared as a decoction (a simmered tea) due to its dense and fibrous nature. This method extracts its medicinal properties effectively. Burdock tea is traditionally used to support digestion, detoxification, and skin health.

Tincture: A tincture of burdock root offers a concentrated liquid form, typically used for its detoxifying and skin-cleansing properties. Tinctures are convenient for those who wish to incorporate burdock into their daily routine.

Capsules or Powder: Burdock root powder is sometimes taken in capsule form, especially when targeting skin issues or as part of a detox regimen. It's a convenient way to obtain its benefits without the strong taste of the root.

Food: In Japanese cuisine, burdock root (known as gobo) is commonly consumed as a vegetable, either sautéed, pickled, or in soups and stews. This provides a nutritious source of fiber and minerals.

External Uses

Skin Wash or Poultice: A decoction of burdock root can be applied to the skin as a wash for acne, eczema, and other skin irritations. It's also used in compresses or poultices to reduce inflammation in arthritic joints and soothe skin conditions.

Salve or Cream: Burdock root extracts are often added to skincare formulations for their anti-inflammatory and soothing effects. These are beneficial for sensitive or inflamed skin, providing relief for eczema, psoriasis, and similar skin issues.

How to Harvest

Roots: Burdock roots are best harvested in the fall of the plant's first year, as this is when they're most nutrient-dense. The roots should be carefully dug up, as they can grow deep into the soil. Once harvested, they can be cleaned, sliced, and dried for long-term storage or roasted for immediate use.

Leaves: While the root is most commonly used, the young leaves can also be harvested and used in small amounts in teas or as poultices, though they are quite bitter.

Burs: Burs, or seed heads, are generally avoided in herbal uses due to their prickly nature but play a role in seed propagation.

Precautions

Allergic Reactions: Burdock is in the Asteraceae family, so people with allergies to daisies or ragweed should use it with caution.

Diuretic Effect: Burdock's mild diuretic properties may interact with other diuretic medications. It's advisable to consult a healthcare provider if taking prescription diuretics.

Pregnancy and Nursing: Although generally safe, burdock root is traditionally avoided during pregnancy and breastfeeding due to its strong detoxifying effects.

Identification: When foraging, be careful not to confuse burdock with Deadly Nightshade (belladonna), as the two plants can look similar when young.

Energetics

In traditional herbalism, burdock is considered cooling and drying, making it useful for conditions associated with heat, inflammation, or excess moisture. Its bitter and slightly sweet taste supports its role as a detoxifying and blood-purifying herb, especially for skin and liver-related imbalances.

Conclusion

Burdock is a powerful herb widely recognized for its blood-purifying, detoxifying, and skin-supporting properties. With its roots playing a prominent role in herbal medicine, burdock is particularly valued for supporting liver and kidney function and addressing skin issues like acne and eczema. Its high antioxidant content also makes it a strong ally in reducing inflammation. Burdock root can be enjoyed as a food, decoction, or tincture, offering diverse ways to integrate this herb's benefits into daily life.

Alfalfa (Medicago sativa)

Common Names:

Alfalfa, Lucerne, Buffalo Herb

Botanical Name:

Medicago sativa

Family: Fabaceae (Legume family)

Type: Perennial herb

Origin: Alfalfa is native to southwestern Asia and the eastern Mediterranean. It's one of the oldest cultivated plants, used as both livestock forage and herbal medicine for thousands of years.

Plant Description

Alfalfa is a resilient, deeply-rooted perennial herb that grows about 3 feet tall. It produces dense clusters of purple flowers and small, clover-like leaves. This plant is highly nutritious, drawing minerals and nutrients from deep in the soil through its extensive root system, and is often used as a "green" superfood.

Key Features

Height: Alfalfa typically grows between 2-3 feet (0.6-0.9 meters).

Leaves: The leaves are small and divided into three leaflets, resembling clover. They are slightly toothed at the edges and are often consumed as a fresh or dried supplement.

Flowers: The flowers are small, purple to lavender, and bloom in clusters. These flowers eventually produce coiled seed pods.

Roots: Alfalfa has a deep root system that can reach up to 20 feet, allowing it to access minerals and moisture from deep in the soil, making it particularly drought-resistant and nutrient-rich.

Medicinal Properties:

Alfalfa is highly regarded for its nutritive, anti-inflammatory, diuretic, digestive-supporting, and cholesterol-lowering properties. It's often used as a tonic to support overall vitality, balance hormones, and aid in detoxification.

Nutritive Tonic: Alfalfa is packed with essential vitamins (A, C, E, and K) and minerals, including calcium, iron, magnesium, and potassium. It's often used as a nourishing herb, especially for those with deficiencies, and can help promote general well-being.

Cholesterol Reduction: Alfalfa has shown promise in helping to reduce cholesterol levels due to its high fiber content and the presence of compounds called saponins. These compounds help remove cholesterol from the bloodstream and prevent its absorption in the body.

Hormone Balance: Alfalfa contains phytoestrogens, plant compounds that mimic estrogen in the body. This can help balance hormones, especially for menopausal women, and is sometimes used to alleviate symptoms like hot flashes and mood swings.

Diuretic: Alfalfa has mild diuretic properties, which aid the body in removing excess fluids and toxins through urination. This action supports kidney health and helps reduce bloating and fluid retention.

Digestive Support: Alfalfa is known to stimulate appetite and improve digestion. The high fiber content promotes bowel regularity, while its alkaline nature can help neutralize stomach acid, reducing symptoms of acid reflux.

Anti-Inflammatory: Alfalfa has anti-inflammatory properties, making it useful for reducing pain and swelling in conditions like arthritis. Its nutrient density also helps repair and strengthen joints and tissues.

Interesting Facts

Root System: Alfalfa's root system is one of the deepest of any cultivated plant, sometimes reaching up to 20 feet into the ground. This enables it to draw minerals from deep soil layers, making it one of the most mineral-rich plants.
Cultural Significance: In Arabic, alfalfa means "father of all foods" due to its rich nutrient profile. It's considered a fundamental herb in many cultures for enhancing overall health.

Culinary Uses

Alfalfa leaves and sprouts are a nutritious addition to a plant-based diet. They have a mild, slightly nutty flavor and can be added to salads, sandwiches, and wraps. Alfalfa is also a popular addition to green smoothies and juices for its dense nutrient profile.

Traditional and Modern Uses

Internal Uses

Tea or Infusion: Alfalfa leaf tea is a popular method for extracting its vitamins and minerals. Often consumed as a tonic, it's considered beneficial for general health and vitality.

Tincture: Alfalfa tinctures offer a concentrated form of the herb, allowing for easy ingestion of its nutrients and supportive properties, especially for those looking for a daily herbal supplement.

Capsules or Powder: Alfalfa is available in powder or capsule form for those who want a nutrient boost without the taste. It's commonly used in green powders or multivitamin formulations to enhance nutrition.

Sprouts: Alfalfa sprouts are commonly added to salads, sandwiches, and smoothies. These fresh sprouts are nutrient-dense and provide enzymes that aid in digestion and enhance nutrient absorption.

External Uses

Poultice: Alfalfa can be made into a poultice to soothe insect bites, minor wounds, and skin irritations. It's cooling and anti-inflammatory when applied topically.

Skin Care: Alfalfa's antioxidant properties make it useful for promoting skin health. Alfalfa extract or powder can be added to facial masks or scrubs to nourish the skin and promote a healthy glow.

How to Harvest

Leaves: Alfalfa leaves can be harvested when the plant reaches full height, typically in mid-spring to early summer. The leaves can be dried and stored for use in teas, capsules, or tinctures.

Sprouts: Alfalfa seeds are commonly sprouted in jars and harvested after a few days. They are an easy and fresh way to enjoy alfalfa's nutrients.

Flowers: While not as commonly used as the leaves or sprouts, the flowers can be harvested and used in teas for added flavor and nutrition.

Precautions

Autoimmune Disorders: Alfalfa contains an amino acid called L-canavanine, which may exacerbate symptoms of lupus and other autoimmune conditions. People with autoimmune issues should consult a healthcare provider before using alfalfa.

Medication Interactions: Alfalfa's vitamin K content may interfere with blood-thinning medications like warfarin. Those on anticoagulants should avoid or limit alfalfa intake.

Pregnancy and Breastfeeding: While generally safe in food amounts, large doses of alfalfa supplements are not recommended during pregnancy or breastfeeding due to its hormonal effects.

Energetics

In traditional herbalism, alfalfa is considered cooling and moistening. Its nutrient-dense profile and mild nature make it a gentle tonic suitable for many constitutions, especially beneficial for those needing nourishment and gentle support for skin, hormones, and digestion.

Conclusion

Alfalfa is a versatile and highly nutritious herb known for its high vitamin and mineral content. Often used as a nourishing tonic, it supports skin health, digestion, hormone balance, and cholesterol levels. Alfalfa is commonly enjoyed in various forms, including tea, tincture, capsules, and as fresh sprouts, making it accessible for a range of health goals. With its gentle action and rich nutritional profile, alfalfa is a valuable herb for promoting overall wellness and vitality.

Mugwort (Artemisia vulgaris)

Common Names:

Mugwort, Common Wormwood, Felon Herb, St. John's Plant

Botanical Name:

Artemisia vulgaris

Family: Asteraceae (Daisy family)

Type: Perennial herb

Origin: Native to Europe, Asia, and North Africa, mugwort has a rich history in traditional herbal medicine and folklore across many cultures, from Europe to Asia.

Plant Description

Mugwort is a hardy perennial herb with tall, bushy growth, and a characteristic silvery underside to its leaves. The plant grows to about 3–6 feet tall and produces small, yellowish to reddish flowers. Known for its slightly bitter, aromatic flavor, mugwort is widely used in traditional medicine, culinary applications, and spiritual practices.

Key Features

Height: Mugwort typically grows between 3–6 feet (1–2 meters).

Leaves: The leaves are deeply lobed, dark green on the top, and silvery-white and downy on the underside. They emit a strong, slightly sage-like aroma when crushed.

Flowers: Mugwort flowers are small and inconspicuous, ranging from yellow to reddish-brown. They bloom in late summer and grow in clusters along the plant's tall, slender stems.

Roots: The root system is fibrous and helps the plant spread easily, allowing it to grow in various conditions, even in poor soils.

Medicinal Properties

Mugwort is known for its digestive, nervine (calming), menstrual-regulating, and antimicrobial properties. It's particularly popular in traditional practices for its role in supporting digestion, enhancing dreams, and balancing the menstrual cycle.

Digestive Aid: Mugwort is a bitter herb that stimulates bile production and aids digestion. It's commonly used for relieving indigestion, bloating, and gas and can stimulate appetite, making it useful in cases of poor appetite or sluggish digestion.

Nervine and Calming Effects: Mugwort has mild calming effects, helping ease anxiety and promote relaxation. It is often used to relieve tension and stress and can be particularly beneficial for nervous stomach issues associated with anxiety.

Menstrual Support: Mugwort has been traditionally used as an emmenagogue, meaning it can help stimulate menstruation. This makes it useful for regulating irregular periods, relieving menstrual cramps, and easing premenstrual symptoms.

Antimicrobial and Antifungal: Mugwort contains essential oils that have antimicrobial and antifungal properties. It's sometimes used in topical applications for treating minor infections and as a natural insect repellent.

Dream Enhancement: Mugwort has a unique reputation as a dream herb, often used to promote vivid dreams, lucid dreaming, and enhanced dream recall. This effect may be due to its impact on the nervous system, providing a gentle calmness that allows for more relaxed sleep and, potentially, vivid dreams.

Culinary Uses

Mugwort has a long history of culinary use in various cultures, particularly in East Asian and European cuisines. The young leaves are used in small quantities to flavor soups, stews, and meat dishes. In Japan, it's known as yomogi and is used in rice cakes and teas. In Europe, it was once used to flavor beer before hops became popular.

Interesting Facts

"Mother Herb": Mugwort is often referred to as a "mother herb" in herbal medicine for its connection to menstrual health and women's reproductive wellness. It's also associated with the moon and was used historically for feminine health.

Dream Herb: Mugwort's use as a dream herb has been documented across many cultures. In European folklore, it was believed to help people experience prophetic or lucid dreams, and it continues to be used by some as an aid for exploring the subconscious.

Traditional and Modern Uses

Internal Uses

Tea or Infusion: Mugwort tea is one of the most popular methods for consuming this herb. It's typically brewed as a digestive aid, mild sedative, or pre-bedtime tea to support dream work.

Tincture: Mugwort tinctures offer a concentrated form, commonly used for menstrual and digestive support. This form allows for easy dosing and storage, making it convenient for long-term use.

Capsules or Powder: Dried mugwort leaves can be ground into a powder and taken in capsules. This is a more convenient way to consume mugwort if the bitter taste of tea is too strong.

External Uses

Moxibustion: In traditional Chinese medicine, dried mugwort is used in a technique called moxibustion, where it's burned near the skin to warm and stimulate specific acupuncture points. This practice is said to enhance the flow of energy or "qi" in the body.

Dream Pillow: Dried mugwort leaves are often added to sachets or dream pillows to support vivid dreaming. Placed under the pillow or near the bed, the scent is thought to enhance dream clarity.

Topical Wash or Compress: A mugwort infusion can be used as a wash or compress for wounds, bug bites, or minor skin irritations. It's also traditionally used for tired, achy feet and as a soothing bath herb.

How to Harvest

Leaves: Mugwort leaves can be harvested throughout the growing season. Harvest young leaves for culinary use or mid-season leaves for medicinal use. The leaves should be dried in a well-ventilated, shaded area to preserve their volatile oils.

Flowers: The flowering tops can be harvested in late summer when the plant is in full bloom. These are typically used for dream work or tinctures.

Roots: While less commonly used, mugwort roots can be harvested in the fall. They are known for their slightly stronger medicinal properties compared to the leaves.

Precautions

Pregnancy: Mugwort should not be used during pregnancy, as it may stimulate uterine contractions. It's generally considered unsafe for pregnant women.

Allergies: Mugwort is in the Asteraceae family, so those with allergies to daisies, ragweed, or chrysanthemums should exercise caution.

Overuse: Excessive consumption of mugwort may cause nausea or stomach upset due to its bitter compounds. It's recommended to use it in moderate doses.

Toxicity: Mugwort contains thujone, a compound that can be toxic in large doses, affecting the nervous system. Regular use should be moderate, and it's generally recommended not to use it continuously.

Energetics

In traditional herbalism, mugwort is considered warming and drying. Its warming nature supports circulation, while its dryness is useful for damp, stagnant conditions, such as bloating and indigestion. Energetically, it's viewed as a grounding and calming herb, helping to center the mind and spirit, especially in practices like meditation and dream work.

Conclusion

Mugwort is a unique herb with a broad range of uses, from supporting digestion and calming the mind to balancing the menstrual cycle and enhancing dreams. Its long history in folklore and spiritual practices makes it popular among herbalists and enthusiasts seeking to connect with both physical and subtle aspects of well-being. Whether used in teas, tinctures, or dream pillows, mugwort provides versatile support, especially for those drawn to its mystical and calming qualities.

Yarrow (Achillea millefolium)

Common Names:

Yarrow, Milfoil, Soldier's Woundwort, Thousand-leaf, Nosebleed Plant

Botanical Name:

Achillea millefolium

Family: Asteraceae (Daisy family)

Type: Perennial herb

Origin: Native to Europe, Asia, and North America, yarrow has been used for centuries in traditional medicine for its wound-healing, anti-inflammatory, and antiseptic properties. Its botanical name honors Achilles, the legendary Greek warrior who reportedly used yarrow to treat his soldiers' wounds.

Plant Description

Yarrow is a hardy perennial herb known for its feathery leaves and clusters of tiny flowers, typically white, though they can also appear in shades of pink, red, and yellow. It commonly grows wild in meadows, along roadsides, and in grassy areas, preferring full sun and well-drained soil.

Key Features

Height: Yarrow typically grows between 1 to 3 feet (30 to 90 cm) tall.

Leaves: The leaves are finely divided and feather-like, giving them a soft, fern-like appearance. This leaf structure contributes to one of its nicknames, "thousand-leaf."

Flowers: Yarrow flowers are small, usually white, and grow in dense clusters at the top of the stems. Each tiny flower head is made up of multiple florets, creating a flat-topped or slightly domed flower cluster.

Aroma: Yarrow has a distinct, earthy scent with slight hints of sweetness and spice, which intensifies when the leaves or flowers are crushed.

Medicinal Properties

Yarrow is known for its anti-inflammatory, antiseptic, antispasmodic, and astringent properties. It is commonly used for wound care, digestive health, menstrual issues, and as a remedy for colds and flu.

Wound Healing and Blood Clotting: Yarrow has been traditionally used as a "woundwort" for its ability to stop bleeding and disinfect wounds. The leaves and flowers contain compounds that encourage blood clotting, and its antiseptic properties help prevent infection. Fresh yarrow leaves can be applied directly to wounds as a poultice to control bleeding and speed healing.

Anti-Inflammatory and Pain Relief: Yarrow contains anti-inflammatory compounds that help reduce pain and swelling in wounds, bruises, and sprains. Its pain-relieving and muscle-relaxing properties make it a popular choice for easing aches, menstrual cramps, and digestive discomfort.

Menstrual Health: Yarrow is considered an effective remedy for menstrual cramps and excessive bleeding. Its astringent and antispasmodic properties help reduce heavy menstrual flow and ease muscle tension, which can relieve cramps. Yarrow tea is commonly used for these purposes and is valued as a uterine tonic.

Digestive Health: Yarrow is a digestive bitter, helping stimulate bile flow and support the digestive process. It can relieve symptoms of indigestion, bloating, and gas. Yarrow also has antispasmodic effects on the digestive tract, making it useful for soothing stomach cramps and easing symptoms of irritable bowel syndrome (IBS).

Cold and Flu Relief: Yarrow is a popular herb for managing colds, fevers, and flu symptoms. It promotes sweating, which helps reduce fevers, and its astringent and anti-inflammatory properties relieve sore throats and congestion. Yarrow tea is often combined with other herbs like elderflower and peppermint for cold and flu relief.

Interesting Facts

Traditional Fever Remedy: Yarrow has been used as a fever-reducing herb since ancient times. It induces sweating, helping to lower body temperature, which is why it's often used during fevers associated with colds and flu.

Symbol of Protection: Yarrow was traditionally thought to have protective qualities. It was used in various rituals and was sometimes planted near homes to ward off evil spirits and negative energy.

How to Harvest

Leaves: Yarrow leaves can be harvested in spring or early summer, before the plant flowers. The younger leaves are milder and easier to use.

Flowers: Yarrow flowers are harvested when they are in full bloom during late spring or summer. They should be dried or used fresh for teas, tinctures, and other remedies.

Storing: Once dried, yarrow leaves and flowers can be stored in an airtight container in a cool, dark place for up to a year.

Precautions

Allergic Reactions: Yarrow belongs to the Asteraceae family, which includes daisies and ragweed. Individuals with allergies to this plant family may experience skin irritation or allergic reactions when using yarrow.

Pregnancy and Nursing: Yarrow may stimulate uterine contractions, so it should not be used by pregnant women. Nursing mothers should also use it with caution and consult a healthcare provider.

Potential Skin Sensitivity: Some people may experience skin irritation from contact with fresh yarrow leaves. Gloves are recommended during harvesting or handling for sensitive skin.

Energetics

In traditional herbalism, yarrow is considered cooling and drying. It helps reduce heat and inflammation in the body, making it beneficial for fevers, wounds, and other conditions associated with excess heat and moisture. It is especially valued for moving "stuck" energy, such as in cases of poor circulation or stagnation.

Conclusion

Yarrow is a versatile herb known for its wound-healing, anti-inflammatory, and astringent properties. From treating minor wounds and infections to supporting menstrual health and easing digestive discomfort, yarrow has a wide range of applications in herbal medicine. It is a cooling and drying herb, useful for managing conditions associated with inflammation, heat, and excess moisture. With a history rooted in folklore and traditional medicine, yarrow continues to be a valuable addition to the herbalist's toolkit for its numerous therapeutic uses.

Raspberry Leaf (Rubus Idaeus)

Common Names:

Raspberry Leaf, Red Raspberry Leaf

Botanical Name:

Rubus Idaeus

Family: Rosaceae (Rose family)

Type: Perennial herbaceous plant

Origin: Native to Europe, Asia, and North America, raspberry plants have been used for centuries, with their leaves highly valued in herbal medicine, especially for women's health.

Plant Description

Raspberry plants are deciduous shrubs with thorny stems, and they produce familiar red, sometimes black or golden, raspberry fruits. The leaves are the part used medicinally and are often dried for use in teas and other preparations.

Key Features

Height: Raspberry bushes grow up to 4–6 feet (1.2–1.8 meters) tall.

Leaves: Raspberry leaves are green, serrated, and slightly rough to the touch. They have a distinctive light underside, giving them a silver-like appearance.

Stems: The plant's stems are woody, thorny, and produce new canes each year.

Flowers and Fruit: Raspberry plants bloom with small white flowers in spring, followed by clusters of edible red or golden berries in the summer.

Medicinal Properties

Raspberry leaf is well-known for its astringent, tonic, anti-inflammatory, and nutritive properties. It is most commonly used to support reproductive health, though it offers benefits for digestion, skin, and general health as well.

Women's Reproductive Health: Raspberry leaf is particularly celebrated as a tonic for the female reproductive system. It is commonly used during pregnancy to tone and strengthen the uterus in preparation for labor, potentially reducing complications and labor duration. Additionally, it can help regulate menstrual cycles, reduce heavy menstrual bleeding, and relieve PMS symptoms due to its astringent and toning effects on the uterus.

Uterine Tonic: Raspberry leaf is considered a "uterine tonic," helping to strengthen the uterine muscles and potentially making labor easier and more efficient. For this reason, it's frequently recommended for use during the second and third trimesters of pregnancy as a tea, though some also use it postpartum to help the uterus return to its pre-pregnancy state.

Digestive Health: Raspberry leaf has mild astringent properties that can soothe the digestive tract, making it helpful for diarrhea and mild digestive discomfort. It can be used to tighten and tone the tissues of the digestive system, which is beneficial for gastrointestinal issues.

Anti-Inflammatory Properties: Raspberry leaf contains anti-inflammatory compounds that are beneficial for soothing inflammation, particularly in the female reproductive organs. This can be especially helpful for women experiencing discomfort from menstrual cramps, endometriosis, and other inflammatory reproductive conditions.

Nutritive Qualities: Raspberry leaf is rich in vitamins and minerals, including vitamins C, E, A, and B, as well as calcium, magnesium, potassium, and iron. These nutrients make it a supportive tonic for overall health, especially during pregnancy when nutritional needs are increased.

Interesting Facts

Rich in Nutrients: Raspberry leaves are nutrient-dense, making them a valuable tonic during pregnancy and times of increased nutritional need. The vitamins and minerals in raspberry leaf are easily absorbed by the body, making it a gentle source of nourishment.

Historical Use in Childbirth: Raspberry leaf has a long-standing reputation as a women's herb, used by midwives for centuries to support healthy pregnancies and ease childbirth. It was often recommended in folk medicine for its supposed ability to strengthen the uterine muscles and prevent complications during labor.

Traditional and Modern Uses

Internal Uses

Tea or Infusion: Raspberry leaf tea is the most common way to use this herb. The dried leaves are steeped in hot water to make a mild, nutritious tea that can be consumed throughout the day. It's often recommended for menstrual and pregnancy support and is used as a general health tonic.

Capsules: Raspberry leaf is available in capsule form for those who prefer a more concentrated or convenient option, especially when taken as part of a daily health regimen.

Tincture: A tincture made from raspberry leaf offers a concentrated liquid form, which can be added to water or taken directly. Tinctures are convenient for those who may not wish to drink tea but still seek the benefits of the herb.

External Uses

Skin Tonic: Raspberry leaf infusions can be used as a natural skin wash for treating minor irritations, redness, and rashes. Its astringent qualities help tone the skin and reduce inflammation.

Mouthwash or Gargle: Raspberry leaf tea can be used as a gargle for sore throats or mouth ulcers. Its astringent and anti-inflammatory properties help soothe inflamed tissues and reduce discomfort.

How to Harvest

Leaves: Raspberry leaves are best harvested in the spring or early summer, just before the plant begins to flower, as this is when they are most nutrient-dense. Leaves should be picked from healthy plants, preferably from young canes.

Drying and Storing: To preserve them, raspberry leaves are dried and stored in an airtight container in a cool, dark place. Dried leaves can last up to a year if properly stored.

Precautions

Pregnancy: Although raspberry leaf is commonly used during pregnancy, it's generally recommended to start during the second or third trimester, as its uterine-toning properties may not be advisable in early pregnancy. Always consult with a healthcare provider before use.

Allergic Reactions: While rare, some people may have an allergy to plants in the Rosaceae family. Discontinue use if any allergic reactions occur.

Excessive Use: While generally safe, excessive consumption can lead to mild digestive upset, so it's best to use raspberry leaf within recommended limits.

Energetics

In traditional herbalism, raspberry leaf is considered cooling and drying. Its astringent properties help to tone and tighten tissues, making it beneficial for conditions of excess moisture or relaxation. Raspberry leaf is a balancing herb, especially for the reproductive and digestive systems, and is often used to restore balance in conditions of excess heat or inflammation.

Conclusion

Raspberry leaf is a well-loved herb in herbal medicine, renowned for its supportive and toning effects on the female reproductive system. With its high content of vitamins and minerals, it also serves as a gentle nutritive tonic, especially valued during pregnancy and for general reproductive health. Known for its cooling, drying, and astringent qualities, raspberry leaf is helpful in conditions that involve inflammation or excess moisture. Widely used as a tea, raspberry leaf is both a comforting daily tonic and a go-to remedy for women's health, particularly during times of transition such as pregnancy, menstruation, and menopause.

Nettle (Urtica dioica)

Common Names:

Nettle, Stinging Nettle, Common Nettle, Greater Nettle

Botanical Name:

Urtica dioica

Family: Urticaceae

Type: Perennial herb

Origin: Native to Europe, Asia, and parts of North America, nettle is found worldwide, thriving in temperate climates, often in moist, nutrient-rich soils. It grows wild along riverbanks, forests, meadows, and disturbed areas like roadsides.

Plant Description

Nettle is a herbaceous perennial that can grow between 2 to 6 feet tall. It is most famous for its stinging hairs (called trichomes) that cover the stems and leaves. These tiny hairs act as a defense mechanism, releasing irritants (such as histamine, formic acid, and acetylcholine) when touched, causing a stinging sensation on contact with the skin.

Key Features

Leaves: The leaves are dark green, heart-shaped with serrated edges, and have a slightly rough texture. They grow opposite on the stems.

Stem: Square and fibrous, sometimes reddish, and covered with stinging hairs.

Flowers: Small, inconspicuous green flowers grow in clusters from the leaf axils. Nettle is dioecious, meaning male and female flowers grow on separate plants.

Roots: Nettle has creeping rhizomes that spread and can form dense patches.

Medicinal Properties

Anti-inflammatory: Nettle has been traditionally used to treat inflammatory conditions, particularly arthritis and joint pain. Its anti-inflammatory compounds help reduce swelling and pain.

Allergy Relief: Nettle is a natural antihistamine and is commonly used to relieve symptoms of hay fever, such as sneezing, itchy eyes, and runny nose. It inhibits histamine receptors, providing allergy relief without the drowsiness of many over-the-counter antihistamines.

Blood Builder: Rich in iron, nettle is used to help treat iron deficiency anemia. The high vitamin C content enhances the absorption of iron, making it an excellent herb for building blood and increasing energy.

Diuretic: Nettle is a natural diuretic, meaning it promotes urination and helps the body excrete excess fluids and toxins. It is often used in herbal remedies to support kidney function and to reduce water retention.

Support for Benign Prostatic Hyperplasia (BPH): Nettle root has been used for centuries to support prostate health, particularly in men with BPH. It helps reduce the symptoms associated with prostate enlargement, such as frequent urination.

Skin and Hair Health: Nettle is often used in natural skincare products to soothe skin irritations like eczema, rashes, and acne. It is also known to stimulate hair growth, improve scalp health, and combat dandruff due to its silica and sulfur content.

Bone Health: With its high calcium and magnesium levels, nettle helps maintain strong bones and teeth. Its silica content also contributes to healthy connective tissues.

Nutritional Content

Nettle is incredibly nutrient-dense, especially in its young, tender leaves. It is often referred to as a "superfood" due to its rich profile of vitamins, minerals, and bioactive compounds.

Vitamins: Rich in vitamins A, C, K, and several B vitamins.
Minerals: Contains high amounts of iron, calcium, magnesium, potassium, and silica.
Other Compounds: Chlorophyll, carotenoids, flavonoids, and tannins are also present, contributing to its antioxidant properties.

Traditional and Modern Uses

Internal Uses

Tea: Nettle leaves are commonly steeped to make tea, which is used to treat a variety of conditions, including allergies, joint pain, and fatigue. The tea is also considered a gentle detoxifier and blood purifier.

Tinctures: Nettle tinctures are made from both the leaves and roots, typically used for more potent doses in supporting prostate health, allergies, and inflammation.

Capsules/Powder: Dried nettle can be encapsulated or ground into powder for easier consumption. The powder can be added to smoothies or foods for a nutrient boost.

External Uses

Hair Rinse: Nettle tea or infused oil is used as a hair rinse to improve scalp health and stimulate hair growth.

Skin Care: Nettle extracts are added to creams or used in poultices to soothe eczema, acne, and other skin conditions.

Culinary Uses

Food: Young nettle leaves are used in cooking after they've been boiled or dried (which neutralizes the sting). They are commonly used in soups, stews, and as a green in dishes similar to spinach. Nettle pesto is another popular dish.

How to Harvest

Harvest young leaves in spring (before the plant flowers) for food or medicine. Once nettle flowers, the leaves develop a gritty texture and are no longer ideal for consumption.

Wear gloves and long sleeves when harvesting to avoid being stung by the plant's tiny hairs.

To reduce the sting, blanch or dry the leaves before handling.

Precautions

Stinging: Handle nettle carefully when fresh to avoid the sting from its trichomes. However, once dried or cooked, the stinging effect is neutralized.

Allergic Reactions: Although rare, some individuals may be allergic to nettle and experience skin irritation or digestive upset.

Interaction with Medications: Nettle may interact with certain medications, such as blood thinners, diuretics, or anti-inflammatory drugs. Consult a healthcare provider before using nettle medicinally if you are on any medication.

Interesting Facts

Fiber Source: Historically, nettle fibers were used to make textiles, ropes, and fishing nets due to their strength and durability.

Insect Repellent: Nettle is used in organic gardening as a natural insect repellent or as a component in liquid fertilizers, benefiting plant growth.

Energetics

In herbalism, nettle is often classified as cooling and drying, meaning it is beneficial for conditions involving heat, excess fluids, or dampness, such as inflammation, swelling, or excessive mucous production.

Conclusion

Nettle (Urtica dioica) is a powerful medicinal herb with a long history of use. Its ability to provide nutrition, support detoxification, alleviate allergies, and reduce inflammation makes it one of the most versatile and valued herbs in both traditional and modern herbal medicine. Whether taken as a tea, tincture, or food, nettle offers a wealth of health benefits.

Chamomile (Matricaria chamomilla or Chamaemelum Nobile)

Common Names:

Chamomile, Roman Chamomile (Chamaemelum Nobile), German Chamomile (Matricaria chamomilla), Ground Apple

Botanical Names:

German Chamomile: Matricaria chamomilla (also known as Matricaria recutita)
Roman Chamomile: Chamaemelum Nobile

Family: Asteraceae (Daisy family)

Type: German Chamomile is an annual herb, while Roman Chamomile is a perennial herb.

Plant Description

Chamomile is a small, fragrant herb with daisy-like flowers, known for its calming and soothing properties. It has been widely used in herbal medicine for thousands of years, often as a remedy for various ailments, including stress, insomnia, digestive issues, and skin conditions. The plant's name comes from the Greek word chamaimelon, meaning "ground apple," referring to the pleasant, apple-like fragrance emitted by the plant, especially when its leaves are crushed.

Key Features

Height: Chamomile typically grows to about 12–24 inches (30–60 cm) tall.

Leaves: The feathery leaves are finely divided, with a soft, green appearance.

Flowers: Chamomile's flowers resemble small daisies, with a yellow cone-shaped center and white petals radiating outward. The flowers are where the majority of the plant's medicinal properties are concentrated.

Roots: Shallow and fibrous, suitable for container planting or garden beds.

Medicinal Properties

Chamomile is valued for its wide range of medicinal benefits. Both German and Roman chamomile share similar uses, but German chamomile is most often used in teas and essential oils due to its higher concentration of active compounds like bisabolol, apigenin, and flavonoids.

Calming and Sedative: Chamomile is famous for its soothing properties, making it an excellent natural remedy for anxiety, stress, and insomnia. Its mild sedative effect can help promote relaxation and better sleep.

Digestive Aid: Chamomile is frequently used to alleviate digestive issues such as indigestion, gas, bloating, and cramping. It can help relax the muscles of the digestive tract, reducing discomfort and promoting digestion.

Anti-inflammatory: The herb is rich in anti-inflammatory compounds like alpha-bisabolol and matricin, which help soothe conditions like arthritis, skin irritations, and other inflammatory disorders.

Antispasmodic: Chamomile helps reduce muscle spasms, making it useful for conditions such as menstrual cramps or irritable bowel syndrome (IBS).

Skin Soothing: Chamomile is often used in creams, lotions, and compresses for skin irritations, burns, eczema, and rashes. Its anti-inflammatory and antimicrobial properties promote healing and reduce redness and swelling.

Immune Support: Chamomile has mild antimicrobial properties, which can help the body fight off minor infections, particularly when used as a tea during colds or flu.

Wound Healing: Due to its antiseptic properties, chamomile can be applied topically to help heal minor cuts, wounds, and sores.

Traditional and Modern Uses

Internal Uses

Tea: Chamomile tea is perhaps the most popular way to consume chamomile. The dried flowers are steeped in hot water to make a calming beverage that aids sleep, soothes digestive issues, and eases anxiety.

Tincture: Chamomile tinctures are made by steeping the flowers in alcohol, which concentrates their medicinal properties. These tinctures can be used for digestive disorders, menstrual cramps, or as a sleep aid.

Infusions and Capsules: Chamomile extracts can be taken as capsules or added to tonics and infusions for a range of health benefits.

External Uses

Skin Care: Chamomile is used in topical creams, ointments, and compresses for treating burns, eczema, psoriasis, rashes, and other skin conditions. It is gentle enough for sensitive skin and can help reduce inflammation and redness.

Baths: Adding chamomile flowers or essential oil to a warm bath can help soothe irritated skin and promote relaxation.

Hair Rinse: Chamomile is often used as a natural hair lightener and conditioner, especially in blonde or light-colored hair.

How to Harvest

German Chamomile: Harvest the flowers in late spring or early summer when they are fully open and dry. Pick the flowers on a sunny day after the morning dew has evaporated for the best quality.

Roman Chamomile: You can also harvest the flowers or cut back the whole plant and use the leaves and stems for teas or essential oil distillation.

Precautions

Allergic Reactions: Chamomile is related to ragweed and other plants in the daisy family (Asteraceae), so individuals allergic to these plants may also be allergic to chamomile.

Pregnancy: Large amounts of chamomile should be avoided during pregnancy due to its mild uterine stimulant effect.

Drug Interactions: Chamomile can interact with blood-thinning medications or sedatives, so consult a healthcare provider if you are taking any medications.

Interesting Facts

Chamomile in Folklore: Chamomile has long been associated with peace, harmony, and healing. In ancient Egypt, chamomile was associated with the sun god Ra, and its flowers were used as offerings and remedies for fever.

Lawn Chamomile: Roman chamomile is sometimes planted as a ground cover or "lawn" due to its pleasant fragrance when walked upon.

Energetics

Chamomile is considered cooling and drying in herbal energetics, making it particularly effective for "hot" conditions such as inflammation, fever, or irritability. It's also calming for the nervous system, digestive system, and skin, helping to relax and soothe without being too overpowering.

Conclusion

Chamomile, whether in its German or Roman form, is a versatile herb with a rich history of medicinal use. Its ability to calm the mind, soothe the stomach, heal the skin, and ease inflammation makes it a staple in herbal medicine. Chamomile tea is one of the most popular herbal teas worldwide, known for its calming effects and gentle support for overall well-being. Whether you use chamomile for its calming tea, its soothing skin applications, or its delicate flavor in culinary creations, this herb offers gentle but powerful support for the body and mind.

Echinacea (Echinacea spp.)

Common Names:

Echinacea, Purple Coneflower, American Coneflower

Botanical Name:

Echinacea purpurea, Echinacea angustifolia, Echinacea pallida (the most commonly used species in herbal medicine)

Family: Asteraceae (Daisy family)

Type: Perennial herb

Origin: Native to North America, particularly the Great Plains. It has been traditionally used by Native American tribes for its powerful medicinal properties. Today, echinacea is widely grown in gardens around the world as both an ornamental plant and a medicinal herb.

Plant Description

Echinacea is a hardy, herbaceous perennial known for its vibrant purple-pink flowers and conical seed heads. It's a drought-resistant plant that thrives in well-drained soil and full sun, making it a popular choice for both medicinal herb gardens and natural landscapes.

Key Features

Height: Echinacea plants typically grow between 2 to 4 feet (60 to 120 cm) tall.

Leaves: The leaves are lance-shaped, dark green, and slightly rough to the touch, growing alternately along the stems.

Flowers: Echinacea flowers are large and daisy-like, with prominent spiny, brown to orange central cones surrounded by purple, pink, or white petals. The cone is a distinguishing feature, giving the plant its name, derived from the Greek word echinos, meaning "hedgehog" or "sea urchin," due to its prickly appearance.

Roots: The roots of echinacea are long, thick, and fibrous, and are often harvested for medicinal use.

Medicinal Properties

Echinacea is best known for its immune-boosting properties. It has been used for centuries to treat infections, promote wound healing, and enhance the body's natural defenses. The herb contains a variety of active compounds, including polysaccharides, flavonoids, alkamides, and phenolic compounds like cichoric acid, which are believed to be responsible for its medicinal effects.

Immune System Support: Echinacea is widely used to enhance immune function. It stimulates the body's immune response, helping to fight off infections such as the common cold, flu, and other respiratory infections. It is often taken at the onset of illness to reduce the duration and severity of symptoms.

Antiviral and Antibacterial: The herb has been shown to have mild antiviral and antibacterial properties, making it useful for combating infections. It is especially effective in supporting the body's natural defenses against viral infections like colds and the flu.

Anti-inflammatory: Echinacea contains compounds that can reduce inflammation, making it useful for treating conditions such as sore throats, swollen lymph nodes, and inflammatory skin issues. Its anti-inflammatory effects also make it beneficial for easing joint pain and other inflammatory conditions like arthritis.

Wound Healing: Traditionally, echinacea was used externally to treat wounds, burns, and insect bites. It promotes healing by enhancing the body's natural defenses and reducing inflammation.

Antioxidant: Echinacea is rich in antioxidants, which help neutralize free radicals in the body, protecting cells from oxidative stress and supporting overall health.

Supports Skin Health: Echinacea's antimicrobial and anti-inflammatory properties make it useful for treating skin conditions such as eczema, acne, and minor wounds. It is sometimes added to skincare products for its healing and soothing effects.

Traditional and Modern Uses

Internal Uses

Tinctures: Echinacea tinctures are one of the most popular ways to use the herb medicinally. Made from the roots, leaves, or flowers, echinacea tinctures are used to stimulate the immune system, fight off infections, and reduce inflammation.

Teas: Echinacea tea is commonly consumed at the first sign of a cold or flu. It can be made from the dried flowers, leaves, and roots. Drinking echinacea tea is a gentle way to boost immunity and reduce the duration of illnesses.

Capsules or Tablets: Echinacea is also available in capsule or tablet form, offering a convenient way to take the herb as a daily immune support or for acute infections.

External Uses

Topical Ointments or Creams: Echinacea is often used in ointments, salves, or creams to treat skin conditions, minor wounds, burns, and insect bites. It helps speed up the healing process and reduce inflammation.

Poultices: The plant's fresh or dried leaves and roots can be made into poultices to apply directly to the skin to treat wounds or insect bites.

How to Harvest

Flowers: Echinacea flowers can be harvested when fully open, usually in mid to late summer. Cut the stems just below the flower heads and hang them to dry for tea or tinctures.

Roots: Harvest echinacea roots in the fall after the plant has gone dormant. Dig up the plant carefully to preserve the thick, fibrous roots. The roots can be used fresh or dried for medicinal preparations.

Precautions

Allergic Reactions: Like other members of the Asteraceae family (daisies), echinacea may cause allergic reactions in some individuals, especially those allergic to ragweed, chrysanthemums, or marigolds.

Autoimmune Conditions: Echinacea stimulates the immune system, so it may not be suitable for people with autoimmune diseases such as lupus or rheumatoid arthritis. Always consult a healthcare professional before use.

Pregnancy and Breastfeeding: While echinacea is generally considered safe, pregnant and breastfeeding women should consult a healthcare provider before taking echinacea supplements.

Energetics

Echinacea is considered cooling and drying in traditional herbal energetics, making it useful for "hot" conditions such as fever, infections, and inflammation. It stimulates the immune system, making it suitable for both preventative and acute care in infections.

Interesting Facts

Native American Medicine: Echinacea was used extensively by Native American tribes for a variety of ailments, including snake bites, wounds, toothaches, and respiratory infections. It was considered a panacea, or cure-all.

Popularity in Modern Herbalism: Echinacea is one of the most well-researched and popular herbs in Western herbal medicine. It is a staple in many herbal medicine cabinets for its ability to prevent and treat colds and infections.

Conclusion

Echinacea is one of the most powerful and well-known herbs for immune system support. Whether used to prevent illness, fight off infections, or soothe inflammation, echinacea offers a wide range of health benefits. With its antiviral, antibacterial, and anti-inflammatory properties, it is a staple in herbal medicine, particularly for those seeking natural ways to boost immunity and overall wellness. Whether taken as a tea, tincture, or topical remedy, echinacea is a trusted ally for health and healing.

Valerian (Valeriana officinalis)

Common Names:

Valerian, Garden Valerian, All-Heal, Setwall

Botanical Name:

Valeriana officinalis
Family: Caprifoliaceae (Honeysuckle family)

Type: Perennial herb

Origin: Native to Europe and parts of Asia, valerian has a long history of use in traditional medicine for its calming and sedative properties. It has since spread to North America and other temperate regions, where it's grown both as an ornamental plant and for its medicinal roots.

Plant Description:

Valerian is a tall, clumping perennial herb with fern-like leaves and fragrant clusters of small, pale pink or white flowers. Its medicinal use primarily comes from the roots, which emit a strong, earthy, somewhat unpleasant odor when dried.

Key Features

Height: Valerian can grow between 4 to 5 feet (1.2 to 1.5 meters) tall.

Leaves: The leaves are divided into lance-shaped leaflets that grow in pairs along the stems. They are bright to dark green, giving the plant a fern-like appearance.

Flowers: Small, fragrant, and typically white or pale pink, valerian flowers bloom in umbrella-shaped clusters at the top of tall stems in mid-summer.

Roots: The most important part of the valerian plant for medicinal use. The roots are thick and fibrous, and when harvested, they emit a strong, musky odor. This is due to the presence of compounds that contribute to its medicinal effects.

Medicinal Properties

Valerian is best known for its ability to promote relaxation, reduce anxiety, and improve sleep. It has been used for centuries as a natural remedy for insomnia, nervous tension, and stress. The root of the plant contains several active compounds, including valerenic acid, valepotriates, and isovaleric acid, which are thought to contribute to its calming effects.

Sedative and Relaxant: Valerian is a natural sedative often used to promote restful sleep and reduce the time it takes to fall asleep. It is commonly taken as a remedy for insomnia, particularly when caused by anxiety or nervous tension.

Anxiety and Stress Relief: Valerian has been used for centuries to ease anxiety and stress. Its mild sedative effects help calm the nervous system, making it useful for those experiencing nervousness, agitation, or stress-related symptoms.

Muscle Relaxant: Valerian has antispasmodic properties, meaning it can help relax tense muscles and alleviate muscle cramps. It is sometimes used to relieve menstrual cramps, muscle spasms, or general tension in the body.

Calms the Nervous System: Valerian works as a nervine, which means it has a calming effect on the nervous system. It is used to ease symptoms of nervous system disorders, such as nervous exhaustion, trembling, or restlessness.

Migraine Relief: Some herbalists use valerian to help alleviate headaches or migraines, particularly those caused by tension or stress. Its ability to relax muscles and reduce nervous tension can help mitigate headache symptoms.

Supports Heart Health: While valerian is primarily used for its calming effects, it also has mild cardiovascular benefits. It can help lower blood pressure in some individuals by reducing stress and promoting relaxation.

Traditional and Modern Uses

Internal Uses

Tinctures: Valerian tinctures are commonly used for their fast-acting sedative effects. Tinctures made from valerian root are taken to calm the nerves, ease anxiety, or help induce sleep.

Capsules and Tablets: Valerian is available in capsule or tablet form, often combined with other relaxing herbs like hops or passionflower. These supplements are used to promote sleep, reduce anxiety, and relieve stress.

Teas: Valerian tea, though not known for its pleasant taste or smell, is another common way to consume the herb. The dried root is steeped in hot water and consumed before bedtime to promote relaxation and improve sleep quality.

External Uses

Poultices: While less common than internal use, valerian root can be used externally in poultices to help with muscle pain, cramps, or to reduce tension in specific areas of the body.

Aromatherapy

Essential Oil: Valerian essential oil is sometimes used in aromatherapy to promote relaxation, alleviate stress, and reduce nervousness. It can be diffused into the air or applied topically after dilution to help calm the mind and body.

How to Harvest

Roots: Valerian root is typically harvested in the fall, after the plant has finished flowering and the leaves have died back. At this time, the roots are at their peak potency. The roots can be dug up, cleaned, and dried for use in teas, tinctures, or capsules.

Precautions

Drowsiness: Valerian is a sedative, so it can cause drowsiness and should not be taken before driving or operating machinery. Some people may feel groggy or experience "valerian hangover" the morning after use.

Individual Sensitivities: While valerian helps many people relax, a small percentage of people may experience the opposite effect, feeling overstimulated or restless after taking it.

Pregnancy and Breastfeeding: Valerian is generally not recommended for use during pregnancy or breastfeeding, as there is limited research on its safety in these populations.

Drug Interactions: Valerian may interact with other sedative medications or alcohol, potentially enhancing their effects. Always consult a healthcare provider before combining valerian with other medications.

Energetics

In traditional herbal energetics, valerian is considered warming and moistening, making it beneficial for cold and dry conditions in the body, such as nervous tension, cold-induced insomnia, or muscular stiffness. Its calming and sedative properties make it useful for people who are "overheated" or overstimulated due to stress or anxiety.

Conclusion

Valerian is one of the most well-known herbs for its sedative and relaxing properties. Whether you struggle with insomnia, anxiety, or muscle tension, valerian can provide natural relief and promote a sense of calm and relaxation. Valerian root has been used for centuries as a remedy for nervous tension and sleep disorders, and modern studies continue to support its effectiveness. Whether taken as a tincture, tea, or capsule, valerian remains a trusted and time-honored herbal ally for those seeking relaxation and improved sleep quality.

Turmeric (Curcuma longa)

Common Names:

Turmeric, Indian Saffron, Haldi

Botanical Name:

Curcuma longa

Family: Zingiberaceae (Ginger family)
Type: Perennial herb

Origin: Turmeric is native to Southeast Asia, particularly India, where it has been cultivated for thousands of years. It plays a prominent role in traditional Ayurvedic and Chinese medicine, as well as in the culinary practices of South Asia.

Plant Description

Turmeric is a perennial, rhizomatous herb, closely related to ginger. Its most valuable part is its bright orange-yellow rhizome (underground stem), which is harvested for both culinary and medicinal use. Above ground, turmeric produces lush, large green leaves, while beneath the surface, its aromatic rhizomes spread out in clusters.

Key Features

Height: Turmeric plants typically grow between 3 to 4 feet (0.9 to 1.2 meters) tall.

Leaves: The broad, lance-shaped leaves are bright green and can grow up to 2 feet long. They are similar in appearance to ginger or banana plant leaves.

Flowers: Turmeric produces pale yellow to white flowers, arranged in spike-like clusters. These flowers emerge from a central stem, though the plant rarely flowers outside its native, tropical environment.

Rhizomes: The most important part of the turmeric plant is its thick, knobby rhizomes, which are bright orange or yellow inside and covered in a rough, brown skin. These rhizomes are harvested for their culinary, medicinal, and dyeing properties.

Medicinal Properties

Turmeric is prized for its potent anti-inflammatory, antioxidant, and antimicrobial properties. The primary active compound in turmeric is curcumin, which has been extensively studied for its numerous health benefits, particularly its ability to combat inflammation and oxidative stress. Beyond curcumin, turmeric contains a variety of other bioactive compounds that contribute to its therapeutic effects.

Anti-inflammatory: Turmeric is best known for its ability to reduce inflammation in the body. It has been used in traditional medicine to treat conditions like arthritis, joint pain, and inflammatory skin disorders. Modern research supports turmeric's effectiveness in reducing chronic inflammation, making it useful for treating inflammatory diseases such as rheumatoid arthritis and inflammatory bowel conditions.

Antioxidant: Curcumin, along with other compounds in turmeric, has powerful antioxidant effects, which help neutralize free radicals and protect the body from oxidative damage. This makes turmeric beneficial for overall cellular health and longevity, as well as for protecting against conditions related to oxidative stress, like heart disease and cancer.

Supports Digestive Health: Turmeric has long been used to treat digestive disorders, including indigestion, bloating, and gas. Its anti-inflammatory and antimicrobial properties make it helpful for soothing the digestive tract, and it is commonly used in Ayurvedic medicine to treat liver and gallbladder issues.

Immune Support: Turmeric's ability to modulate the immune system makes it useful for fighting infections and boosting overall immune health. It is often used to help prevent or treat colds, flu, and other infections by enhancing the body's natural defenses.

Promotes Heart Health: Turmeric has been shown to support heart health by improving circulation, reducing cholesterol levels, and preventing the oxidation of LDL cholesterol (a key factor in heart disease). Its anti-inflammatory and antioxidant properties also help protect against damage to the cardiovascular system.

Supports Joint Health: Turmeric is commonly used to treat arthritis and other joint conditions. Its ability to reduce inflammation and oxidative stress helps alleviate pain and improve mobility in people suffering from conditions like osteoarthritis and rheumatoid arthritis.

Skin Health: Turmeric is also used externally for its antimicrobial and anti-inflammatory properties. It is applied topically to treat wounds, acne, eczema, and other skin conditions. Turmeric masks and creams are popular in skincare for their ability to brighten the skin and promote a healthy complexion.

Traditional and Modern Uses

Internal Uses

Powder: Turmeric powder, made from dried and ground rhizomes, is the most common way to consume turmeric. It is widely used in cooking, especially in curries, soups, and teas, and is also taken as a supplement in capsules or tablets for its medicinal benefits.

Teas and Golden Milk: Turmeric tea, often combined with black pepper and ginger, is used to enhance digestion, support the immune system, and reduce inflammation. Golden milk, made with turmeric, milk (or plant-based milk), and spices, is a traditional Ayurvedic drink used to promote overall health and well-being.

Tinctures and Capsules: Turmeric tinctures and capsules provide a more concentrated dose of curcumin, making them popular options for people using turmeric as a natural anti-inflammatory or antioxidant supplement.

External Uses

Poultices: Turmeric paste or poultices are applied to wounds, cuts, and insect bites to promote healing and reduce inflammation. Its antimicrobial properties also help prevent infections.

Facial Masks: Turmeric is a popular ingredient in skincare, used in masks to brighten the complexion, reduce acne, and treat skin disorders such as eczema or psoriasis.

Topical Creams and Salves: Turmeric-infused creams and salves are used to relieve joint pain and muscle soreness, especially for people suffering from arthritis or inflammation.

How to Harvest

Rhizomes: Turmeric rhizomes are typically harvested 9 to 10 months after planting, once the leaves begin to turn yellow and die back. The rhizomes are dug up, cleaned, boiled, and then dried. After drying, they can be ground into powder or used fresh for cooking and medicinal purposes.

Precautions

Staining: Turmeric can stain clothing, countertops, and skin due to its strong yellow pigment. Care should be taken when handling the fresh or powdered herb.

Stomach Upset: Although generally considered safe, consuming large amounts of turmeric may cause stomach upset or gastrointestinal discomfort in some individuals.

Gallbladder Issues: Turmeric stimulates bile production, so people with gallstones or bile duct obstruction should consult a healthcare provider before using turmeric.

Pregnancy: While turmeric is generally considered safe in culinary amounts during pregnancy, concentrated forms (such as supplements or tinctures) should be used with caution, as turmeric may stimulate uterine contractions.

Energetics

In traditional Ayurvedic medicine, turmeric is considered warming and drying, making it useful for conditions characterized by coldness or dampness in the body, such as sluggish digestion, cold-induced joint pain, or congestion. Its bitter and pungent qualities help to stimulate digestion and improve circulation.

Conclusion

Turmeric is one of the most powerful and versatile herbs in both traditional and modern herbal medicine. With its potent anti-inflammatory, antioxidant, and antimicrobial properties, turmeric is valued for treating a wide range of conditions, from joint pain and digestive issues to skin problems and infections. Whether used in cooking, as a supplement, or in topical preparations, turmeric offers immense health benefits. This vibrant yellow herb continues to be a staple in both the kitchen and the medicine cabinet for its ability to promote overall health and well-being.

St. John's Wort (Hypericum perforatum)

Common Names:

St. John's Wort, Tipton's Weed, Goatweed, Klamath Weed

Botanical Name:

Hypericum perforatum

Family: Hypericaceae (St. John's Wort family)

Type: Perennial herb

Origin: Native to Europe, North Africa, and parts of Asia, St. John's Wort has since spread to many parts of the world, including North America. It has a long history of use in traditional herbal medicine, especially for treating mood disorders and skin conditions.

Plant Description

St. John's Wort is a hardy, herbaceous perennial known for its vibrant yellow flowers and medicinal properties. It typically grows in sunny locations like fields, roadsides, and disturbed areas, making it both common and easy to cultivate. The plant's name originates from its traditional harvest time around St. John's Day (June 24) in Christian tradition.

Key Features

Height: St. John's Wort typically grows between 1 to 3 feet (30 to 90 cm) tall, with a bushy, upright habit.

Leaves: The leaves are small, oval-shaped, and opposite, with a characteristic feature: tiny, translucent dots (glands) that can be seen when the leaves are held up to the light, giving them a "perforated" appearance.

Flowers: Bright yellow flowers with five petals grow in clusters at the ends of the branches. Each flower has a profusion of stamens and is around 1 inch (2.5 cm) wide. The flowers bloom in late spring and summer.

Stems: The stems are woody at the base, and the upper part is green, often tinged red. The stems have a distinctive two-edged or ridged structure.

Medicinal Properties

St. John's Wort has been used for centuries, primarily for its effects on the nervous system. It is known for its ability to elevate mood and is often used as a natural remedy for mild to moderate depression, anxiety, and sleep disturbances. The plant's medicinal properties are attributed to its active compounds, including hypericin and hyperforin, which are believed to affect neurotransmitter activity in the brain.

Mood Enhancement and Antidepressant: St. John's Wort is most famous for its use in treating mild to moderate depression. Studies suggest that the active compounds in the herb help balance neurotransmitters like serotonin, dopamine, and norepinephrine, which can elevate mood and improve emotional well-being. It is often used as a natural alternative to conventional antidepressants, especially in Europe.

Anti-Anxiety: St. John's Wort can help reduce anxiety and ease nervous tension. Its ability to calm the nervous system makes it beneficial for people suffering from stress-related conditions, including generalized anxiety disorder and seasonal affective disorder (SAD).

Sleep Aid: By balancing mood and reducing anxiety, St. John's Wort also aids in improving sleep quality. It can be used to treat insomnia, particularly when sleeplessness is linked to emotional stress or mild depression.

Wound Healing and Anti-Inflammatory: St. John's Wort has a long history of external use for wound healing, burns, and inflammation. The herb's anti-inflammatory and antimicrobial properties make it effective for treating minor cuts, bruises, and skin irritations. It is also used in ointments and oils to alleviate nerve pain, such as sciatica and neuralgia.

Antiviral: Some studies suggest that St. John's Wort has antiviral properties, particularly against viruses like herpes simplex. This has led to its use in certain traditional treatments for viral infections.

Pain Relief: St. John's Wort oil is commonly used for topical pain relief, especially for nerve-related pain. It is often applied to alleviate discomfort from conditions like sciatica, neuralgia, or muscle pain.

Traditional and Modern Uses

Internal Uses

Tinctures and Extracts: St. John's Wort tinctures and extracts are popular for treating mood disorders, such as mild depression and anxiety. These concentrated forms provide a more potent dose of the herb's active compounds and are typically taken in small, measured amounts.

Teas: While less concentrated than tinctures, St. John's Wort tea can also help improve mood and alleviate anxiety. The dried flowers and leaves are steeped in hot water and consumed regularly for emotional support.

Capsules and Tablets: Standardized St. John's Wort supplements are widely available in capsule or tablet form. These are often used for their antidepressant and anti-anxiety effects and provide a controlled dose of hypericin and hyperforin.

External Uses

St. John's Wort Oil: The infused oil of St. John's Wort is commonly used for external application. It is made by steeping the fresh flowers in oil, usually olive or sunflower oil, for several weeks. The resulting bright red oil is applied topically to treat wounds, burns, bruises, and nerve pain. It is particularly beneficial for soothing sunburns and reducing inflammation in sore muscles.

Salves and Creams: St. John's Wort is often used in herbal salves or creams designed to speed up the healing of wounds and relieve skin conditions like eczema or psoriasis. Its anti-inflammatory properties make it useful for soothing irritation and promoting skin regeneration

How to Harvest

Flowers: The flowers of St. John's Wort are harvested when they are in full bloom, usually around midsummer (near St. John's Day). The flowers are handpicked and can be used fresh or dried for later use.

Leaves and Stems: The leaves are also harvested at the same time as the flowers. Both the leaves and flowers can be dried and stored for making teas, tinctures, and oils.

Precautions

Photosensitivity: One of the most well-known side effects of St. John's Wort is photosensitivity. When taken in high doses, the herb can make the skin more sensitive to sunlight, increasing the risk of sunburn and rashes, especially in fair-skinned individuals.

Drug Interactions: St. John's Wort can interact with a variety of medications, including antidepressants, birth control pills, blood thinners, and immunosuppressants. It may reduce the effectiveness of these drugs or cause adverse reactions. Always consult a healthcare provider before using St. John's Wort, especially if you are on prescription medications.

Pregnancy and Breastfeeding: St. John's Wort is generally not recommended during pregnancy or breastfeeding due to a lack of research on its safety in these populations.

Energetics

In herbal energetics, St. John's Wort is considered warming and drying. It is used to alleviate conditions associated with coldness and stagnation, such as depressive moods, sluggish digestion, and slow wound healing. Its warming nature makes it useful for promoting circulation and improving energy levels.

Conclusion

St. John's Wort is one of the most widely recognized herbs for its antidepressant and mood-enhancing properties. Whether used internally as a tincture, tea, or capsule to treat mild depression and anxiety, or externally as an oil for wound healing and pain relief, it offers a range of benefits. With a long history in traditional medicine, this vibrant yellow-flowered plant continues to be a natural remedy for supporting emotional well-being, reducing inflammation, and soothing the nervous system. However, due to its potential for drug interactions and side effects, it should be used with care and under professional guidance.

Ginger (Zingiber officinale)

Common Names:

Ginger, Ginger Root, Sheng Jiang (in Traditional Chinese Medicine)

Botanical Name:

Zingiber officinale

Family: Zingiberaceae (Ginger family)

Type: Perennial herb

Origin: Ginger is native to Southeast Asia and has been cultivated for over 5,000 years. It plays a significant role in traditional medicine systems like Ayurveda, Traditional Chinese Medicine, and folk medicine around the world, especially in tropical and subtropical regions.

Plant Description

Ginger is a herbaceous perennial that grows from rhizomes, which are thick underground stems used for both culinary and medicinal purposes. The ginger plant thrives in warm, humid climates and is widely grown in India, China, Southeast Asia, and Africa. It is known for its pungent, spicy flavor and potent medicinal properties.

Key Features

Height: Ginger plants can grow 2 to 4 feet (0.6 to 1.2 meters) tall, forming a leafy clump.

Leaves: Ginger leaves are long, narrow, and lance-shaped, growing in alternating patterns along the stems. They can reach up to 12 inches (30 cm) in length and are dark green.

Flowers: The plant occasionally produces yellow-green flowers with purple bases. The flowers are tubular and grow from spikes that arise directly from the rhizome.

Rhizomes: The rhizome, often referred to as the "root," is thick, gnarled, and light brown on the outside with a pale yellow to creamy white interior. The rhizome's strong aroma and flavor are its most distinctive features.

Medicinal Properties

Ginger is valued for its warming, stimulating, and anti-inflammatory properties. It has been used for thousands of years to treat a wide range of ailments, particularly those related to digestion, inflammation, and circulation. The bioactive compounds in ginger, especially gingerol, shogaol, and zingerone, contribute to its therapeutic effects.

Anti-Inflammatory: Ginger is renowned for its ability to reduce inflammation. The compound gingerol, in particular, has powerful anti-inflammatory effects that can help alleviate conditions like arthritis, joint pain, and muscle soreness. It's commonly used to reduce pain and swelling in both acute injuries and chronic inflammatory conditions like osteoarthritis.

Digestive Aid: One of ginger's most famous uses is as a digestive tonic. It stimulates digestion, relieves nausea, and helps with bloating, gas, and indigestion. Ginger is often used to treat motion sickness, morning sickness during pregnancy, and nausea related to chemotherapy. It also supports the digestive system by increasing bile production and promoting gut motility.

Antioxidant: Ginger contains potent antioxidants that help combat oxidative stress and neutralize harmful free radicals in the body. This makes ginger beneficial for supporting overall cellular health and protecting against conditions related to aging and oxidative damage, such as heart disease and cancer.

Immune Booster: Ginger is known for its ability to boost the immune system and protect against infections. Its antimicrobial properties can help fight off respiratory infections, colds, and flu. Ginger also has warming qualities that help improve circulation and promote sweating, which can assist the body in eliminating toxins.

Antimicrobial: The antimicrobial properties of ginger make it useful for preventing bacterial and viral infections. Ginger is particularly effective in fighting oral bacteria linked to conditions like gingivitis and periodontitis.

Circulation and Heart Health: Ginger stimulates circulation, making it useful for cold hands and feet, and helps to thin the blood, which may reduce the risk of blood clots and improve cardiovascular health. Some studies suggest that ginger can help lower cholesterol levels and blood pressure, further supporting heart health.

Pain Relief: Ginger is effective in reducing various types of pain, including headaches, migraines, and menstrual cramps. It can be used both internally and externally to relieve discomfort. Ginger's warming effect can ease sore muscles and joint stiffness when applied topically as a poultice or in a bath.

Traditional and Modern Uses

Internal Uses

Teas and Infusions: Ginger tea, made by steeping fresh or dried ginger in hot water, is one of the most popular ways to use ginger. It is commonly consumed to relieve nausea, improve digestion, and soothe cold or flu symptoms. Ginger can be combined with other herbs like lemon, honey, or turmeric to enhance its effects.
Tinctures: Ginger tinctures provide a concentrated form of the herb and are used to treat nausea, improve circulation, or reduce inflammation. A few drops of ginger tincture can be added to water or tea for quick relief from digestive discomfort or cold symptoms.
Capsules and Tablets: Ginger supplements are available in capsule or tablet form and are often used for chronic inflammatory conditions, digestive support, or to alleviate motion sickness. Ginger supplements provide a convenient way to take higher doses of gingerol and other active compounds.
Powder: Ground ginger powder is a common kitchen spice but also a medicinal preparation. It can be mixed into food, smoothies, or beverages to aid digestion and provide anti-inflammatory benefits.

External Uses

Poultices: A ginger poultice, made from fresh grated ginger, can be applied topically to relieve sore muscles, joint pain, or stiffness. It is particularly effective for treating arthritis, muscle sprains, or back pain due to its warming properties.
Ginger Baths: Adding fresh or powdered ginger to a warm bath can help relax muscles, improve circulation, and promote detoxification through sweating.
Inhalation: Ginger can be used in steam inhalations to relieve congestion, coughs, and other respiratory issues. The warming, antimicrobial properties of ginger make it effective for clearing sinuses and soothing the throat.

How to Harvest

Rhizomes: Ginger is typically harvested 8 to 10 months after planting. The rhizomes are carefully dug up, cleaned, and either used fresh or dried for later use. The younger ginger rhizomes (harvested earlier) have a milder flavor and are more tender, while older rhizomes are spicier and tougher.

Precautions

Blood Thinning: Ginger has mild blood-thinning properties, which can be beneficial for cardiovascular health, but it may also increase the risk of bleeding when taken with anticoagulant medications (such as warfarin). People taking blood thinners should consult a healthcare provider before using large amounts of ginger.

Stomach Sensitivity: While ginger is great for digestion, consuming it in excess may irritate the stomach or cause heartburn in some individuals, especially those prone to acid reflux.

Pregnancy: Ginger is often recommended for nausea during pregnancy, but it should be used in moderation. While it is considered safe in small amounts, higher doses should be avoided during pregnancy without consulting a healthcare provider.

Energetics

In traditional herbal medicine, ginger is considered warming and stimulating. It is used to counteract coldness in the body, support digestion, and improve circulation. It is especially beneficial in conditions associated with cold, sluggish digestion, or poor circulation.

Culinary Uses

Ginger is widely used in cooking, particularly in Asian and Indian cuisines. It adds a warm, spicy flavor to dishes and is commonly used in stir-fries, soups, curries, and baked goods. Ginger is also a key ingredient in beverages like ginger ale, ginger beer, and various herbal teas. Fresh ginger can be grated or sliced into dishes, while dried or powdered ginger is used for seasoning.

Conclusion

Ginger is one of the most versatile and widely used medicinal herbs, known for its warming, stimulating, and anti-inflammatory properties. It has been used for thousands of years in traditional medicine systems to treat a wide variety of ailments, including digestive issues, inflammation, pain, and respiratory infections. Whether used as a tea, tincture, or poultice, ginger offers potent therapeutic benefits for both internal and external conditions. Its culinary uses only enhance its value, making it a staple ingredient in kitchens and herbal medicine cabinets worldwide.

Ashwagandha (Withania somnifera)

Common Names:

Ashwagandha, Indian Ginseng, Winter Cherry

Botanical Name:

Withania somnifera

Family: Solanaceae (Nightshade family)

Type: Perennial herb

Origin: Ashwagandha is native to India, North Africa, and parts of the Middle East. It has been used in Ayurvedic medicine for over 3,000 years as a powerful adaptogen, helping the body resist physical and mental stress. Ashwagandha is also used in Unani and African traditional medicine for various health conditions.

Plant Description

Ashwagandha is a hardy, drought-resistant plant that thrives in arid and semi-arid regions. It's typically grown in sandy, well-drained soils and can tolerate poor soil conditions. The name "Ashwagandha" comes from the Sanskrit words "ashva," meaning horse, and "gandha," meaning smell, referring to the strong odor of the root, which is said to smell like a horse. The plant's association with strength and vitality mirrors the properties it provides.

Key Features

Height: Ashwagandha plants grow between 1.5 to 5 feet (0.5 to 1.5 meters) tall, forming a bushy, shrub-like structure.

Leaves: The leaves are dull green, ovate, and about 2 to 6 inches (5 to 15 cm) long. They have a smooth texture and are alternately arranged along the stems.

Flowers: Small, pale green or yellow flowers bloom in clusters at the base of the leaves. They are bell-shaped and inconspicuous.

Fruits: The fruit is a small, round, bright red berry enclosed in a papery calyx, similar in appearance to a tiny tomato or ground cherry.

Roots: The roots of the Ashwagandha plant are thick, tuberous, and light brown. These roots are the most commonly used part of the plant in herbal medicine.

Medicinal Properties

Ashwagandha is primarily known as an adaptogen, a type of herb that helps the body adapt to stress and promotes overall balance and resilience. Its active compounds, including withanolides, alkaloids, and steroidal lactones, are responsible for many of its health benefits. It has a wide range of therapeutic uses, particularly in reducing stress, boosting vitality, and enhancing cognitive function.

Adaptogenic and Anti-Stress: Ashwagandha is renowned for its ability to reduce stress, anxiety, and fatigue. By regulating the body's stress hormone levels (especially cortisol), it helps improve mental clarity and emotional resilience. In Ayurveda, it's considered a rasayana, or rejuvenator, promoting overall health and longevity. Regular use helps combat the physical and mental toll of chronic stress.

Energy and Vitality: Ashwagandha enhances stamina and energy, making it ideal for individuals dealing with chronic fatigue or those needing a vitality boost. It is often referred to as the "Indian ginseng" due to its energy-boosting effects, although it doesn't act as a stimulant. It works by improving the body's natural energy production and supporting healthy mitochondrial function.

Cognitive Function: The neuroprotective properties of Ashwagandha help improve memory, focus, and overall cognitive function. It is believed to promote brain cell regeneration and reduce oxidative damage to the brain. As a result, Ashwagandha is commonly used as a nootropic (brain-boosting herb) and has been studied for its potential to prevent or slow neurodegenerative conditions like Alzheimer's and Parkinson's disease.

Immune Support: Ashwagandha boosts the immune system by promoting the production of white blood cells and improving overall immune response. It is often used to support recovery from illness and to increase resistance to common infections. In Ayurveda, it is also used as a tonic to strengthen the immune system after a prolonged illness or period of stress.

Anti-Inflammatory and Antioxidant: Ashwagandha's anti-inflammatory properties help reduce swelling, pain, and inflammation associated with chronic conditions like arthritis and autoimmune diseases. Its antioxidants also protect the body from oxidative stress and reduce the damage caused by free radicals, which contributes to the aging process and the development of diseases like cancer and heart disease.

Hormonal Balance: Ashwagandha helps balance hormones, especially in relation to thyroid and adrenal health. It has been shown to support healthy thyroid function, whether in cases of hypothyroidism (underactive thyroid) or hyperthyroidism (overactive thyroid). It is also used to support adrenal health and reduce symptoms of adrenal fatigue caused by chronic stress.

Reproductive Health: Traditionally, Ashwagandha has been used to enhance sexual health and fertility. In men, it is known to improve sperm count, motility, and testosterone levels, while in women, it helps regulate menstrual cycles and balance reproductive hormones. It has been used in Ayurvedic medicine as an aphrodisiac and to treat sexual dysfunction in both men and women.

Traditional and Modern Uses

Internal Uses

Powder (Churna): Ashwagandha powder is one of the most common forms of the herb. It can be mixed into warm milk, water, or smoothies. In Ayurveda, Ashwagandha powder is traditionally taken with honey or ghee for better absorption and to balance its taste. It is often consumed daily for stress relief, energy enhancement, and overall vitality.

Capsules and Tablets: Ashwagandha is also available in standardized capsules or tablet form for easy and consistent dosing. These are commonly used for stress reduction, improved sleep, and cognitive support.

Tinctures: Ashwagandha tinctures provide a concentrated form of the herb and are usually taken in small amounts. They are beneficial for quick absorption and are often used to treat stress-related conditions and adrenal fatigue.

Teas and Infusions: While less common, Ashwagandha root can be boiled and consumed as a tea. It is often combined with other adaptogenic herbs like holy basil or licorice for a synergistic effect.

External Uses

Ashwagandha Oil: Ashwagandha root is sometimes infused in oil for external application, particularly in Ayurvedic massage. The oil is used to nourish the skin, soothe sore muscles, and promote relaxation. Ashwagandha oil is particularly useful for relieving joint pain, inflammation, and muscle tension.

Topical Pastes: In some traditional practices, Ashwagandha root powder is made into a paste and applied to the skin to treat boils, ulcers, and wounds. It is believed to promote healing and reduce inflammation.

How to Harvest

Roots: The roots of the Ashwagandha plant are harvested when the plant is about one year old. After harvesting, the roots are washed, sliced, and dried for use in powders, tinctures, or teas. They are often sun-dried to preserve their potency.

Precautions

Pregnancy and Breastfeeding: Ashwagandha is not recommended during pregnancy as it may induce contractions and could lead to miscarriage. Nursing mothers should also avoid it unless advised by a healthcare provider.

Autoimmune Conditions: Since Ashwagandha stimulates the immune system, individuals with autoimmune diseases (such as lupus, rheumatoid arthritis, or multiple sclerosis) should use it with caution and under the guidance of a healthcare provider.

Sedative Effects: In some people, Ashwagandha can have a sedative effect, especially when taken in large doses. It's important to be mindful of this, especially if combining Ashwagandha with other sleep aids or medications that affect the nervous system.

Interesting Facts

Modern Research: In recent years, scientific studies have validated many of Ashwagandha's traditional uses, particularly its effects on reducing stress and anxiety, improving sleep, and boosting cognitive function. It has become one of the most studied and popular adaptogens in the West.

Energetics

In Ayurvedic medicine, Ashwagandha is considered warming and nourishing. It is classified as a rasayana (rejuvenator), promoting longevity and vitality. It helps balance Vata and Kapha doshas, making it particularly useful for individuals with Vata imbalances, which manifest as anxiety, nervousness, and dryness.

Conclusion

Ashwagandha is a potent adaptogen that has been revered for thousands of years for its ability to balance the body, reduce stress, and promote vitality. Whether used to enhance energy, relieve anxiety, support cognitive function, or balance hormones, Ashwagandha offers a wide range

Milk Thistle (Silybum marianum)

Common Names:

Milk Thistle, Saint Mary's Thistle, Holy Thistle, Marian Thistle

Botanical Name:

Silybum marianum

Family: Asteraceae (Daisy family)

Type: Biennial or annual herb

Origin: Milk thistle is native to Mediterranean regions of Europe, North Africa, and the Middle East, though it is now found throughout the world. It has been used medicinally for over 2,000 years, particularly for liver health and detoxification.

Plant Description

Milk thistle is a robust and spiny plant known for its striking appearance and medicinal properties. It is often grown in warm, sunny climates and thrives in poor, dry soils. The plant's name comes from the white "milky" sap that its leaves release when broken, and the characteristic white veins on the leaves, which according to legend were the Virgin Mary's milk drops.

Key Features

Height: Milk thistle grows between 2 to 6 feet (0.6 to 1.8 meters) tall, with sturdy, upright stems.

Leaves: The leaves are large, deeply lobed, and shiny green with white marbling or veins. They have spiny edges, giving them a thistle-like appearance.

Flowers: The plant produces purple to reddish-pink, thistle-like flowers that bloom from late spring to early summer. These flowers are large and globe-shaped, with spiny bracts surrounding them.

Seeds: The medicinal part of the plant is the seeds, which form after the flowering period. The seeds are small, hard, and shiny brown with a tuft of white hairs (pappus) attached, similar to dandelion seeds.

Medicinal Properties

Milk thistle is best known for its hepatoprotective (liver-protecting) properties. The primary active compound in milk thistle is silymarin, a complex of flavonoids that includes silibinin, silydianin, and silychristin. These compounds have powerful antioxidant, anti-inflammatory, and detoxifying effects, especially for the liver.

Liver Protection and Detoxification: Milk thistle is most famous for its ability to support liver health. It helps protect the liver from toxins, including alcohol, environmental pollutants, and medications like acetaminophen that can cause liver damage. Silymarin works by stabilizing the membranes of liver cells, preventing toxins from entering and aiding in the regeneration of damaged liver tissue. It is commonly used to treat liver conditions such as hepatitis, cirrhosis, and fatty liver disease.

Antioxidant Properties: Silymarin is a powerful antioxidant that helps neutralize harmful free radicals in the body. By reducing oxidative stress, it helps protect cells from damage and slows the aging process. This makes milk thistle beneficial not only for the liver but also for overall cellular health and skin health.

Anti-Inflammatory Effects: Milk thistle has potent anti-inflammatory properties, helping to reduce inflammation both in the liver and throughout the body. Chronic inflammation is a key factor in many degenerative diseases, including heart disease, diabetes, and arthritis. By lowering inflammation, milk thistle may help protect against these conditions.

Gallbladder Support: Milk thistle also supports gallbladder health by promoting the production and flow of bile. This helps the body break down fats and aids in digestion. For this reason, milk thistle is sometimes used to prevent gallstones and improve overall digestive function.

Skin Health: Due to its antioxidant and anti-inflammatory properties, milk thistle can also benefit the skin. It helps protect the skin from damage caused by free radicals, UV exposure, and environmental toxins, potentially slowing the aging process and promoting clearer, healthier skin.

Blood Sugar Regulation: Some research suggests that milk thistle may help improve insulin sensitivity and lower blood sugar levels, making it potentially beneficial for people with type 2 diabetes. Silymarin has been shown to reduce oxidative stress in the pancreas, where insulin is produced, and improve the regulation of blood glucose.

Cholesterol and Heart Health: Milk thistle may also support heart health by lowering cholesterol levels. Silymarin helps reduce LDL (bad) cholesterol and improve HDL (good) cholesterol levels, reducing the risk of heart disease. Its antioxidant and anti-inflammatory effects also protect blood vessels from damage, which contributes to better cardiovascular health.

Traditional and Modern Uses

Internal Uses

Capsules and Tablets: Milk thistle supplements in capsule or tablet form are among the most popular ways to take the herb. These supplements are typically standardized to contain a specific amount of silymarin, making them effective for liver detoxification and support.

Tinctures: Milk thistle tinctures offer a concentrated liquid form of the herb, which can be taken in small amounts with water or tea. Tinctures are often used for liver detox protocols and to support liver regeneration after exposure to toxins or after heavy alcohol consumption.

Powder: Milk thistle seeds can be ground into a fine powder and added to smoothies, teas, or other beverages. This is a convenient way to incorporate milk thistle into daily routines for liver support and antioxidant benefits.

Teas: Milk thistle tea is made from the seeds, leaves, or flowers of the plant. It can be consumed regularly as a gentle way to support liver health and improve digestion.

External Uses

Skin Applications: Milk thistle extract is sometimes used in skincare products due to its antioxidant and anti-inflammatory properties. It helps protect the skin from environmental stressors and can promote healing in cases of acne, eczema, or sun damage.

Poultices: In traditional herbal medicine, milk thistle leaves were sometimes used in poultices to treat skin wounds or infections due to their mild antimicrobial properties.

How to Harvest

Seeds: The seeds are harvested after the flowers have bloomed and died back. Once the seed heads are dry, they can be carefully cut from the plant and stored. The seeds are then cleaned and dried for medicinal use in tinctures, capsules, or powders.

Precautions

Allergies: Milk thistle is a member of the Asteraceae family, which includes ragweed, daisies, and chrysanthemums. People who are allergic to these plants may also experience allergic reactions to milk thistle.

Drug Interactions: Milk thistle can interact with certain medications, especially those that are processed by the liver, such as statins, blood thinners, and certain cancer medications. If you are taking prescription medications, consult a healthcare provider before using milk thistle.

Estrogenic Effects: Milk thistle may have mild estrogen-like effects, so people with hormone-sensitive conditions, such as breast or ovarian cancer, should use it cautiously and under medical supervision.

Energetics

In traditional herbal medicine, milk thistle is considered cooling and drying. It is particularly beneficial for individuals with excess heat or inflammation, especially in the liver or digestive system. Milk thistle is used to clear heat, reduce stagnation, and support detoxification processes in the body.

Culinary Uses

While milk thistle is primarily known for its medicinal properties, the young leaves can be eaten in salads or cooked as a leafy green. The roots and flower heads are also edible, though they are more commonly used in traditional or folk preparations than in modern cuisine.

Conclusion

Milk thistle is one of the most well-known and widely used herbs for liver health, thanks to its powerful hepatoprotective and antioxidant properties. Whether used to protect the liver from toxins, promote detoxification, or reduce inflammation, milk thistle provides a variety of health benefits. Its rich history in both traditional and modern herbal medicine continues to make it a popular choice for those seeking to support their liver, detoxify the body, and improve overall health.

Tinctures

Tinctures are concentrated herbal extracts made by soaking herbs in alcohol, glycerin, or vinegar to extract their active compounds. They offer a potent and convenient way to use herbs for therapeutic purposes. Tinctures are generally taken by dropper in small doses and are favored for their long shelf life and ease of use. Below are detailed examples of various tinctures, their properties, and ideas for use.

★Consult a doctor before consumption

General Tips for Tincture Use

Dilution: Tinctures are typically taken by adding drops to a small amount of water, juice, or tea.

Consistency: For chronic conditions or ongoing support (such as mood stabilization or immune boosting), tinctures should be taken consistently for a few weeks to experience their full effects.

Alcohol-Free Options: If you want to avoid alcohol, glycerin or apple cider vinegar can be used as a base for making alcohol-free tinctures, though the potency may differ slightly.

Ideas for Combining Tinctures

Immune Boosting Tonic: Combine echinacea tincture with elderberry tincture to create a potent immune-supporting tonic. This blend can be taken during cold and flu season for added protection.

Stress Relief Combo: A mixture of ashwagandha and chamomile tinctures creates a calming and grounding blend that can be taken daily for managing stress and anxiety.

Digestion Aid: Combine ginger, peppermint, and fennel tinctures for a powerful digestive aid that can soothe nausea, indigestion, and bloating after meals.

Anti-Inflammatory Mix: A blend of turmeric, ginger, and black pepper tinctures can enhance anti-inflammatory effects, useful for joint pain, arthritis, or general inflammation.

The standard ratio for making herbal tinctures depends on whether you're using fresh or dried herbs, and it also considers the strength of the alcohol used.

For Fresh Herbs

Herb to alcohol ratio: 1:2
Explanation: Use 1 part fresh herb (by weight) to 2 parts alcohol (by volume).
Example: If you have 100 grams of fresh herb, you would use 200 milliliters of alcohol.

For Dried Herbs

Herb to alcohol ratio: 1:5
Explanation: Use 1 part dried herb (by weight) to 5 parts alcohol (by volume).
Example: If you have 100 grams of dried herb, you would use 500 milliliters of alcohol.

Alcohol Strength

40–60% alcohol (80–120 proof) is the most common for most herbs. Vodka or brandy works well.
Higher alcohol (up to 95%) is used for extracting resins or tougher plant materials like roots and barks.

Here's a step-by-step guide for making a tincture using fresh herbs, using the common 1:2 ratio (1 part fresh herb by weight to 2 parts alcohol by volume):

Ingredients and Supplies

Fresh herbs (e.g., basil, lavender, or echinacea)

Alcohol (40–60% alcohol, such as vodka or brandy)

A glass jar with a tight-fitting lid

Measuring scale (to weigh the herbs)

Measuring cup (for alcohol)

Cheesecloth or a fine mesh strainer

Dark glass dropper bottles for storage

A label and pen (for marking the tincture)

Step-by-Step Instructions

Prepare the Fresh Herbs

Harvest the herbs: Use freshly harvested herbs or ones bought from a trusted source. Make sure they are clean, free from dirt, and ideally harvested when they are most potent (for example, in the morning).

Chop or crush the herbs: Chop the herbs finely or lightly bruise them to help release their active compounds.

Weigh the Fresh Herbs

Use a kitchen scale to measure the weight of your fresh herbs.

Example: If you have 100 grams of fresh herbs, this will guide your alcohol measurement in the next step

Measure the Alcohol

Using the 1:2 ratio, you'll need twice the amount of alcohol by volume as the weight of the fresh herbs.

Example: For 100 grams of fresh herbs, you'll need 200 milliliters of alcohol (vodka or brandy).

Choose alcohol that is at least 40% alcohol by volume (80 proof). Vodka and brandy are common choices. Avoid flavored alcohols or those with added sugars.

Combine Herbs and Alcohol in a Jar

Place the fresh herbs into a clean, dry glass jar.

Pour the measured alcohol over the herbs, ensuring that the herbs are fully submerged.

Tip: If the herbs float to the top, use a clean spoon to press them down so they are fully covered by the alcohol. This helps prevent mold growth.

Seal and Label the Jar

Secure the lid tightly to prevent air from getting in.

Label the jar with the name of the herb, the alcohol used, the date, and the ratio (e.g., "Basil Tincture, Vodka, 1:2, November 4, 2024").

This information will help you track the tincture's progress and remember the specifics for future use.

Steep for 4-6 Weeks

Place the jar in a cool, dark location (such as a cupboard or pantry) to let the tincture infuse.

Shake the jar daily to help the extraction process and keep the herbs submerged.

Strain the Tincture

After 4–6 weeks, strain the mixture using cheesecloth or a fine mesh strainer into a clean glass bowl or measuring cup.

Squeeze the herbs to extract as much liquid as possible.

Bottle and Store

Transfer the strained tincture into dark glass dropper bottles for long-term storage. Dark glass helps protect the tincture from light, which can degrade the active compounds.

Label the bottles with the tincture name, alcohol, date, and ratio.

Dosage and Use

Tinctures are potent, so they're usually taken in small amounts, typically 20–40 drops (1–2 droppers full) diluted in water, juice, or tea, depending on the herb and intended use.

Storage: Keep the tincture bottles in a cool, dark place. Tinctures made with alcohol have a long shelf life, typically lasting 1–3 years or more if stored properly.

Here's a step-by-step guide for making a tincture using dried herbs. For dried herbs, the common ratio is 1:5 (1 part dried herb by weight to 5 parts alcohol by volume), as dried herbs are more concentrated than fresh herbs.

Ingredients and Supplies

Dried herbs (e.g., chamomile, echinacea, or valerian root)

Alcohol (40–60% alcohol, such as vodka or brandy)

A glass jar with a tight-fitting lid

Measuring scale (to weigh the herbs)

Measuring cup (for alcohol)

Cheesecloth or a fine mesh strainer

Dark glass dropper bottles for storage

Label and pen (for marking the tincture)

Step-by-Step Instructions

Prepare the Dried Herbs

Measure the dried herbs: Weigh out the dried herbs using a kitchen scale.

Example: If you have 50 grams of dried herbs, this will determine the amount of alcohol needed (see the next step).

Measure the Alcohol

Using the 1:5 ratio, you'll need five times the amount of alcohol by volume as the weight of the dried herbs.

Example: For 50 grams of dried herbs, you would need 250 milliliters of alcohol (vodka or brandy).

Choose alcohol that is at least 40% alcohol by volume (80 proof). Vodka or brandy are common choices because of their neutral flavor and high alcohol content. Avoid flavored alcohols, as they may interfere with the tincture's properties.

Combine Herbs and Alcohol in a Jar

Place the dried herbs into a clean, dry glass jar.

Pour the alcohol over the herbs, ensuring that all the herbs are fully submerged.

Tip: Make sure the herbs stay fully immersed in the alcohol. If they float to the top, use a clean spoon to push them down.

Seal and Label the Jar

Seal the jar tightly with a lid.

Label the jar with important details: the name of the herb, the type of alcohol used, the date, and the herb-to-alcohol ratio (e.g., "Chamomile Tincture, Vodka, 1:5, November 4, 2024").

This ensures you can track the tincture's progress and keep a record for future use.

Steep for 4-6 Weeks

Store the jar in a cool, dark place (like a pantry or cupboard) to allow the herbs to steep and infuse into the alcohol.

Shake the jar daily to help with the extraction process and to keep the herbs submerged in the alcohol.

Strain the Tincture

After 4–6 weeks, strain the herb mixture using cheesecloth or a fine mesh strainer into a clean glass bowl or measuring cup.

Squeeze the herbs to extract as much liquid as possible. You can wrap the herbs in the cheesecloth and press them with a spoon to get the remaining tincture.

Strain the Tincture

After 4–6 weeks, strain the herb mixture using cheesecloth or a fine mesh strainer into a clean glass bowl or measuring cup.

Squeeze the herbs to extract as much liquid as possible. You can wrap the herbs in the cheesecloth and press them with a spoon to get the remaining tincture.

Dosage and Use

Tinctures are potent, and typically only small amounts are needed. The usual dosage is 20–40 drops (1–2 droppers full) diluted in water, tea, or juice, depending on the herb and intended use. Storage: Store the tincture bottles in a cool, dark place. Tinctures made with alcohol have a long shelf life, often lasting 1–3 years or more if stored properly.

Example of a Dried Herb Tincture

Chamomile Tincture

Use 50 grams of dried chamomile flowers.
Measure 250 milliliters of vodka (5 times the weight of the herbs).
Follow the steps above to create a chamomile tincture for calming nerves, aiding sleep, and soothing digestion.

Tips

Consistency: Shake the jar daily to ensure even extraction.
Alcohol-Free Options: If you prefer not to use alcohol, you can substitute glycerin or apple cider vinegar, though these tinctures may be less potent and have a shorter shelf life.
Strength Variations: You can adjust the herb-to-alcohol ratio for a stronger or weaker tincture. For example, a 1:4 or 1:3 ratio would result in a stronger tincture.

Here's a step-by-step guide for making a tincture using roots. Roots often require a stronger alcohol solution or a longer extraction time due to their tough nature, but the process is similar to that of other herbal tinctures. The standard ratio for roots is 1:5 (1 part root by weight to 5 parts alcohol by volume) when using dried roots, or 1:2 when using fresh roots.

Ingredients and Supplies

Fresh or dried roots (e.g., dandelion root, valerian root, or ginger)

Alcohol (typically 40–60% alcohol, like vodka or grain alcohol)

A glass jar with a tight-fitting lid

Measuring scale (to weigh the roots)

Measuring cup (for alcohol)

Cheesecloth or a fine mesh strainer

Dark glass dropper bottles for storage

Label and pen (for marking the tincture)

Step-by-Step Instructions for Making a Root Tincture:

Prepare the Roots

Clean and chop the fresh roots: If you're using fresh roots, wash them thoroughly to remove dirt and debris. Chop them into small pieces to increase the surface area and make it easier for the alcohol to extract the medicinal compounds.
For dried roots: No need to clean, just measure out the required amount.
Example: If using 50 grams of dried root or 100 grams of fresh root, this will guide how much alcohol you need (explained below).

Measure the Alcohol

For dried roots, use a 1:5 ratio (1 part root by weight to 5 parts alcohol by volume).
Example: For 50 grams of dried root, use 250 milliliters of alcohol.
For fresh roots, use a 1:2 ratio (1 part fresh root by weight to 2 parts alcohol by volume).
Example: For 100 grams of fresh root, use 200 milliliters of alcohol.
Alcohol strength: For tough roots, it's often best to use stronger alcohol (40–60% alcohol, such as vodka or brandy), but for particularly resinous or hard roots, some people use 70–95% alcohol (grain alcohol) for better extraction.

Combine the Roots and Alcohol in a Jar

Place the chopped or dried roots into a clean glass jar.

Pour the measured alcohol over the roots, ensuring they are fully submerged. Roots, especially dried ones, may initially float, but they will settle down as they absorb the liquid.

Tip: Make sure the roots are fully covered by alcohol to prevent spoilage or mold formation.

Seal and Label the Jar

Seal the jar tightly with a lid to keep air out.

Label the jar with the details, including the type of root, the alcohol used, the ratio (e.g., "Dandelion Root Tincture, Vodka, 1:5, November 4, 2024").

This helps you track when the tincture was made and remember the ratios for future use.

Steep for 6-8 Weeks

Roots typically take longer to extract fully, so leave the jar in a cool, dark place for 6–8 weeks to allow the alcohol to pull out all the active compounds.

Shake the jar daily to help the extraction process and keep the roots evenly distributed in the alcohol.

Strain the Tincture

After 6–8 weeks, strain the mixture using a fine mesh strainer or cheesecloth into a clean glass container.

Squeeze the roots to extract as much of the liquid as possible. You can use the cheesecloth to wrap the roots and press them to get the remaining tincture out.

Bottle and Store

Transfer the strained tincture into dark glass dropper bottles for storage. The dark glass protects the tincture from light, helping to preserve its potency.

Label the bottles with the name of the root, alcohol type, ratio, and date.

Dosage and Use

Tinctures made from roots are generally strong, and the recommended dosage is typically 20–40 drops (1–2 droppers full) diluted in water, tea, or juice. However, dosage varies depending on the specific root and its medicinal properties.

Storage: Keep the tincture bottles in a cool, dark place. Tinctures made with alcohol can last 1–3 years or longer if stored properly.

Example of a Root Tincture:

Valerian Root Tincture

Ingredients: Dried valerian root (Valeriana officinalis), vodka (40% alcohol)

Steps

Measure 50 grams of dried valerian root.
Add 250 milliliters of vodka (1:5 ratio).
Seal and shake daily for 6–8 weeks.
Strain, bottle, and label as "Valerian Root Tincture, 1:5, Vodka, November 4, 2024."

Uses: Valerian tincture is commonly used as a sleep aid or to reduce anxiety.

Dandelion Root Tincture

Ingredients: Fresh dandelion root (Taraxacum officinale), vodka

Steps

Measure 100 grams of fresh dandelion root.
Add 200 milliliters of vodka (1:2 ratio).
Steep for 6–8 weeks, then strain, bottle, and label.
Uses: Dandelion root tincture is commonly used to support liver health and digestion.

Tips

Longer steeping time: Roots often need a longer extraction period (up to 8 weeks) compared to leaves and flowers, so be patient for the best results.

Alcohol-Free Option: If you prefer to avoid alcohol, you can make a glycerin-based tincture (known as a glycerite) using the same ratios, though glycerites may have a shorter shelf life and slightly reduced potency.

Stronger Alcohol for Resinous Roots: If using resin-rich roots like certain medicinal barks or roots (e.g., myrrh, goldenseal), consider using a higher proof alcohol (70–95%) for better extraction.

Making a tincture from roots allows you to harness their powerful, slow-releasing properties for long-term health benefits. Roots like dandelion, burdock, or valerian can be excellent for digestive health, detoxification, or stress relief, depending on the herb you choose.

Ideas for Combining Tinctures

Immune Boosting Tonic: Combine echinacea tincture with elderberry tincture to create a potent immune-supporting tonic. This blend can be taken during cold and flu season for added protection.

Stress Relief Combo: A mixture of ashwagandha and chamomile tinctures creates a calming and grounding blend that can be taken daily for managing stress and anxiety.

Digestion Aid: Combine ginger, peppermint, and fennel tinctures for a powerful digestive aid that can soothe nausea, indigestion, and bloating after meals.

Anti-Inflammatory Mix: A blend of turmeric, ginger, and black pepper tinctures can enhance anti-inflammatory effects, useful for joint pain, arthritis, or general inflammation.

General Tips for Tincture Use:

Dilution: Tinctures are typically taken by adding drops to a small amount of water, juice, or tea.

Consistency: For chronic conditions or ongoing support (such as mood stabilization or immune boosting), tinctures should be taken consistently for a few weeks to experience their full effects.

Alcohol-Free Options: If you want to avoid alcohol, glycerin or apple cider vinegar can be used as a base for making alcohol-free tinctures, though the potency may differ slightly.

Tinctures are a versatile, effective way to incorporate herbs into daily life, offering concentrated plant medicine in just a few drops. By experimenting with different herbs and combinations, you can create customized tinctures to support your unique health and wellness needs.

★Consult a doctor before consumption

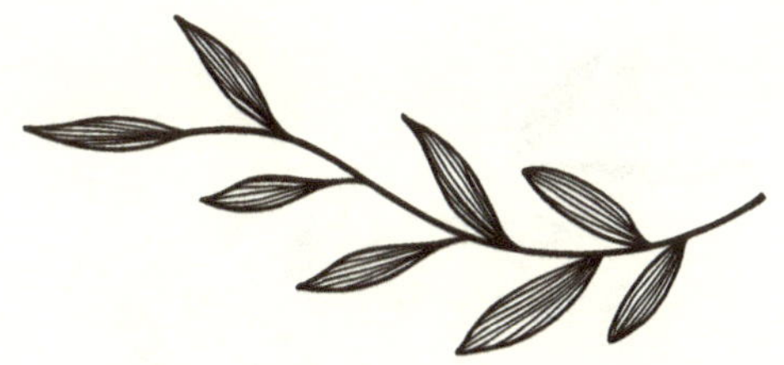

Dandelion Tincture

Ingredients: Dandelion root and leaves, 80-100 proof vodka

Preparation: Use fresh or dried dandelion root and leaves. Chop and fill a glass jar about halfway with the herb. Cover with vodka, seal tightly, and store in a dark place for 4-6 weeks, shaking every few days.

Properties and Uses: Dandelion is known for its detoxifying properties, especially for liver support. It's a mild diuretic, aiding in flushing toxins and supporting kidney health. It also promotes healthy digestion and can help balance skin by supporting liver function.

Dosage: 1-2 ml, 2-3 times daily, diluted in water.

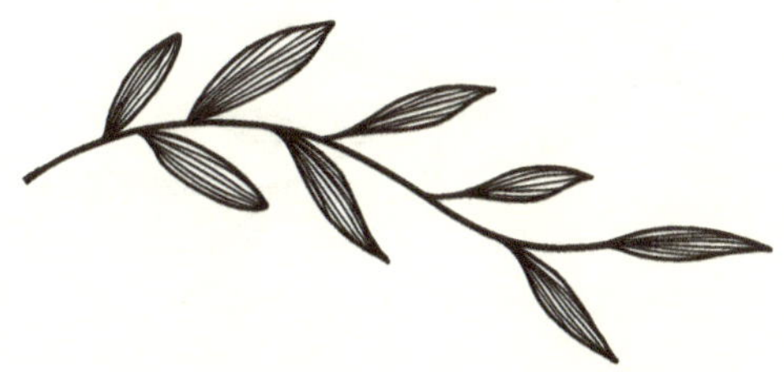

Elderberry Tincture

Ingredients: Dried elderberries, 80-100 proof vodka

Preparation: Fill a jar halfway with dried elderberries, then cover completely with vodka. Let sit for 4-6 weeks, shaking regularly. Strain and bottle the liquid.

Properties and Uses: Elderberry is known for its immune-boosting and antiviral properties, making it excellent for cold and flu season. It's rich in antioxidants and vitamins that support overall immune health.

Dosage: 1-2 ml, 2-3 times daily at the onset of cold symptoms, or daily for immune support.

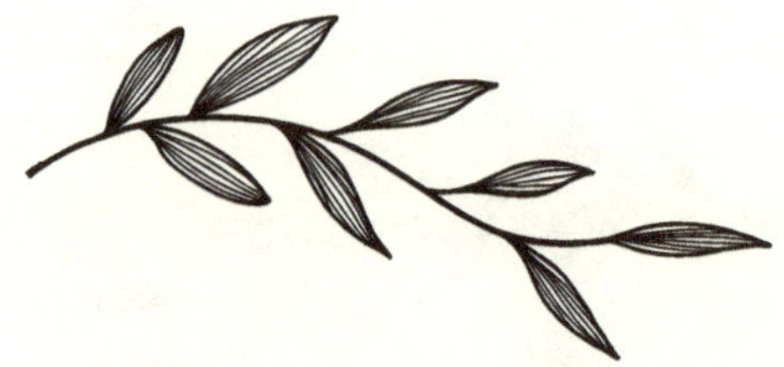

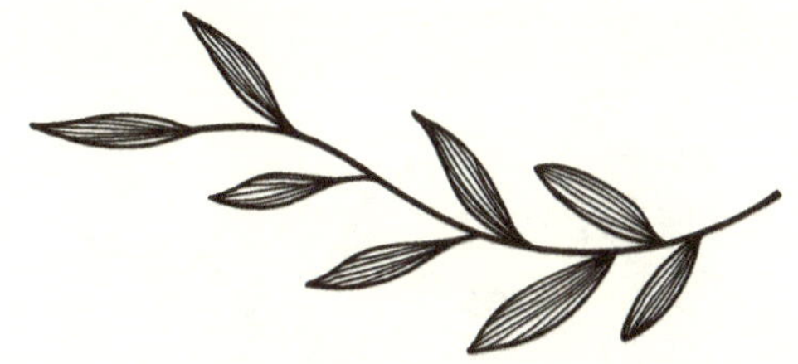

Mullein Tincture

Ingredients: Dried mullein leaves and/or flowers, 80-100 proof vodka

Preparation: Place mullein leaves and flowers in a jar, fill with vodka, and cover tightly. Store in a cool, dark place for 4-6 weeks. Strain and bottle.

Properties and Uses: Mullein is traditionally used as a respiratory herb, helping to soothe coughs, reduce mucus, and relieve lung congestion. It's also mild and safe for children and the elderly.

Dosage: 1-2 ml, 2-3 times daily, especially during respiratory discomfort.

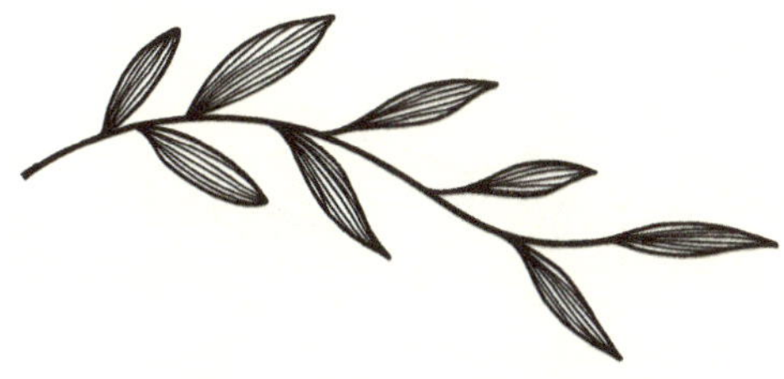

Burdock Root Tincture

Ingredients: Fresh or dried burdock root, 80-100 proof vodka

Preparation: Fill a jar with chopped burdock root, then cover with vodka. Let steep for 4-6 weeks. Strain and transfer to a dropper bottle.

Properties and Uses: Burdock root is a strong blood purifier, helping to detoxify the body. It supports liver function, reduces inflammation, and promotes clear skin. It's also used for lymphatic health.

Dosage: 1-2 ml, 2-3 times daily as a general tonic or for skin and liver health.

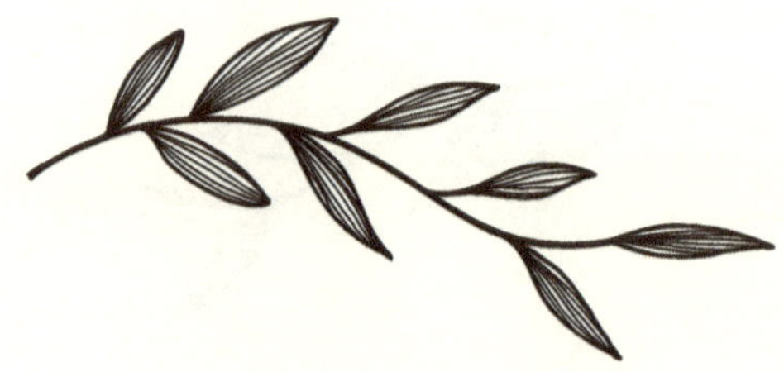

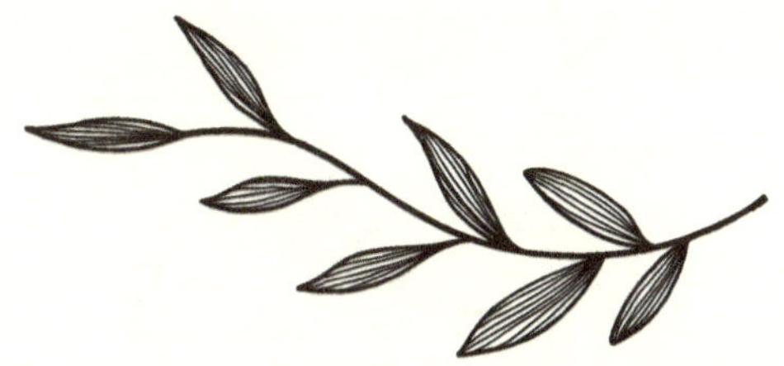

Alfalfa Tincture

Ingredients: Dried alfalfa leaves, 80-100 proof vodka

Preparation: Place dried alfalfa leaves in a jar and cover with vodka. Steep for 4-6 weeks, shaking every few days. Strain and store in a dropper bottle.

Properties and Uses: Alfalfa is nutrient-dense and rich in vitamins A, C, E, and K. It's used as a general tonic for vitality and supports digestion, hormonal balance, and immune health.

Dosage: 1-2 ml, 2-3 times daily for a nutrient boost or as a general wellness tonic.

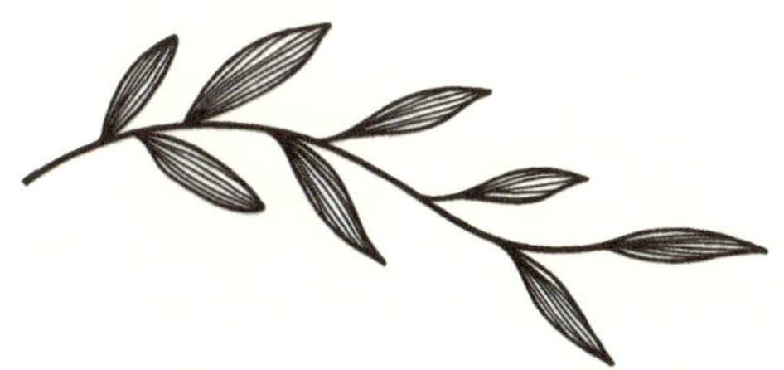

Mugwort Tincture

Ingredients: Fresh or dried mugwort leaves, 80-100 proof vodka

Preparation: Fill a jar with mugwort leaves and cover with vodka. Steep for 4-6 weeks, then strain and bottle.

Properties and Uses: Mugwort is known for its effects on digestion, menstrual health, and dream enhancement. It helps stimulate digestion and is often used for menstrual irregularities. Mugwort is also used traditionally to promote vivid dreaming.

Dosage: 1-2 ml, 1-2 times daily; take before bed if using for dream enhancement.

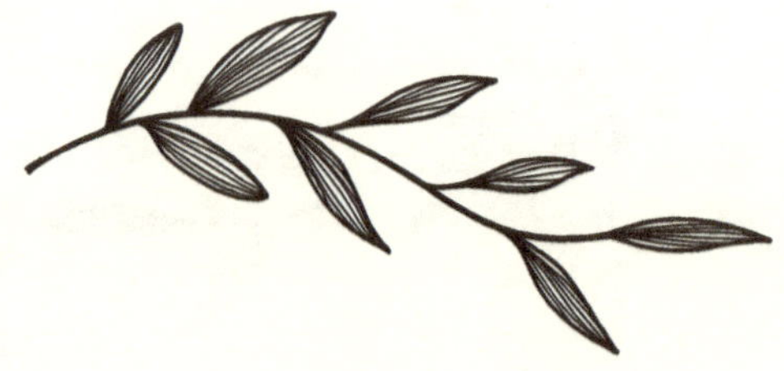

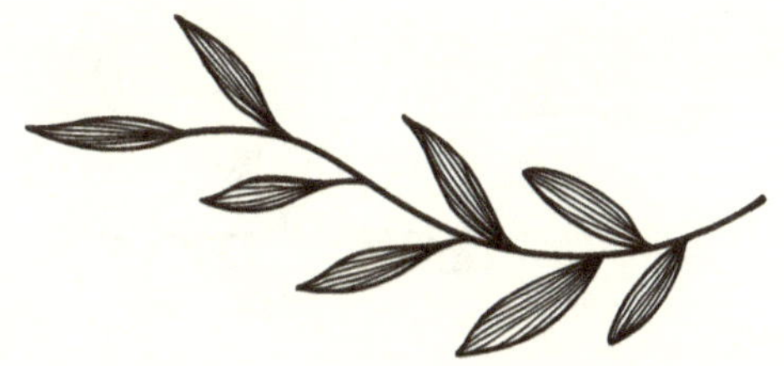

Yarrow Tincture

Ingredients: Fresh or dried yarrow flowers and leaves, 80-100 proof vodka

Preparation: Fill a jar with yarrow flowers and leaves, cover with vodka, and let sit for 4-6 weeks. Shake regularly, then strain and bottle.

Properties and Uses: Yarrow has anti-inflammatory, astringent, and antimicrobial properties. It supports immune health, can reduce fevers, and helps with wound healing. It's also useful for digestive issues and can aid circulation.

Dosage: 1-2 ml, 2-3 times daily as a general tonic or during illness.

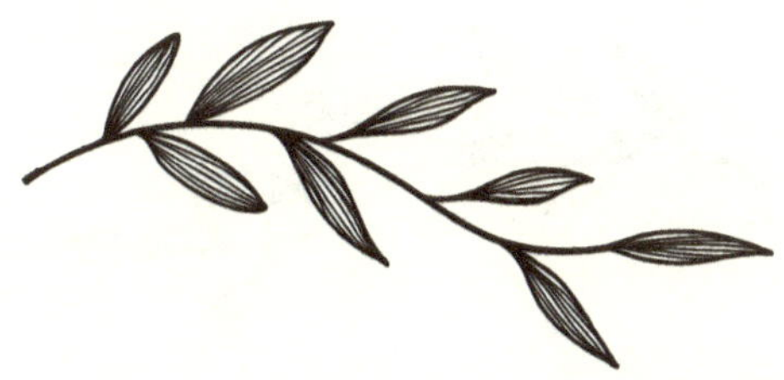

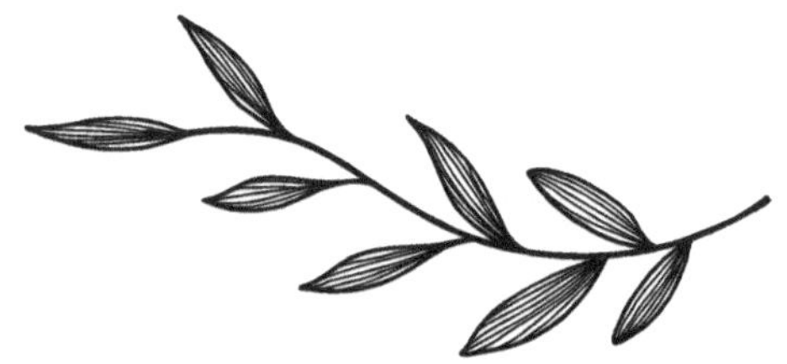

Raspberry Leaf Tincture

Ingredients: Dried raspberry leaves, 80-100 proof vodka

Preparation: Fill a jar halfway with raspberry leaves, cover with vodka, and let steep for 4-6 weeks. Strain and transfer to a dropper bottle.

Properties and Uses: Raspberry leaf is known for its high mineral content, especially iron, and its ability to tone the uterus. It's commonly used to support women's reproductive health, particularly during pregnancy, and can ease menstrual cramps.

Dosage: 1-2 ml, 2-3 times daily; during pregnancy, consult a healthcare professional before use.

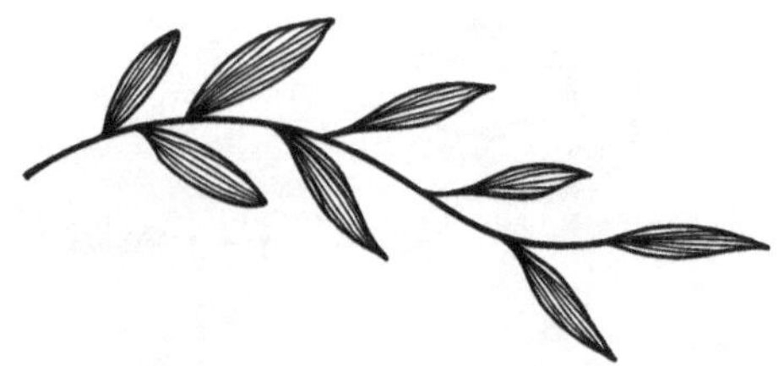

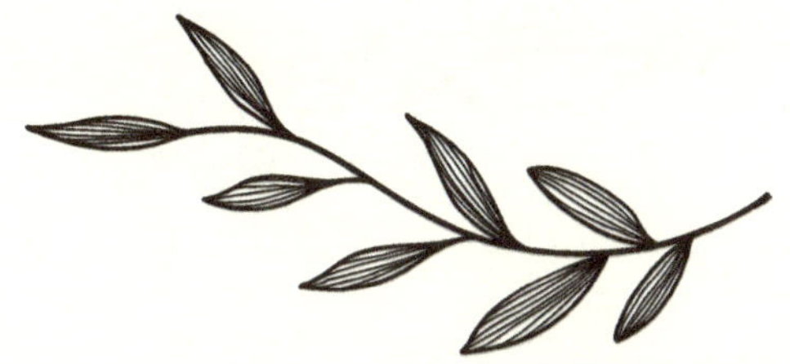

Nettle Tincture

Ingredients: Fresh or dried nettle leaves, 80-100 proof vodka

Preparation: Place nettle leaves in a jar and cover with vodka. Let sit in a cool, dark place for 4-6 weeks. Strain and store.

Properties and Uses: Nettle is highly nourishing, rich in vitamins and minerals, especially iron. It's used for allergy relief, as an anti-inflammatory, and as a general health tonic. Nettle also supports kidney function and is beneficial for skin and hair health.

Dosage: 1-2 ml, 2-3 times daily, particularly during allergy season or as a daily tonic.

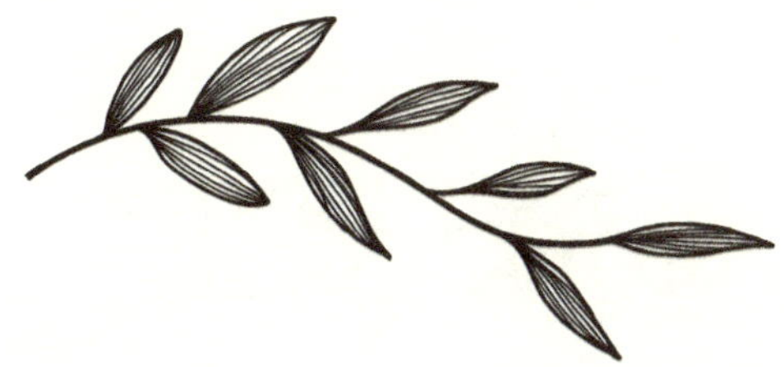

Chamomile Tincture

Ingredients: Dried chamomile flowers (Matricaria chamomilla), alcohol (vodka or brandy).

Process: Chamomile flowers are soaked in alcohol for 4–6 weeks. Chamomile's active compounds, such as flavonoids and volatile oils, are extracted, offering soothing and anti-inflammatory properties.

Uses: Chamomile tincture is known for its calming effects, making it ideal for reducing stress, anxiety, and promoting restful sleep. It can also be used to ease digestive discomfort, such as indigestion or bloating, and to soothe inflammation.

Dosage: 20–30 drops in a small glass of water or tea before bedtime or when needed for relaxation.

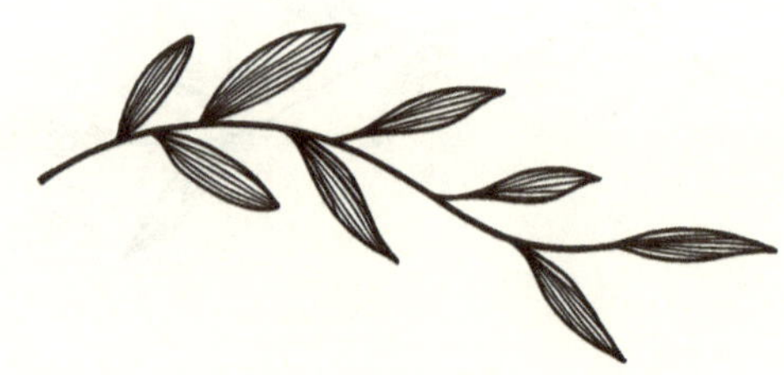

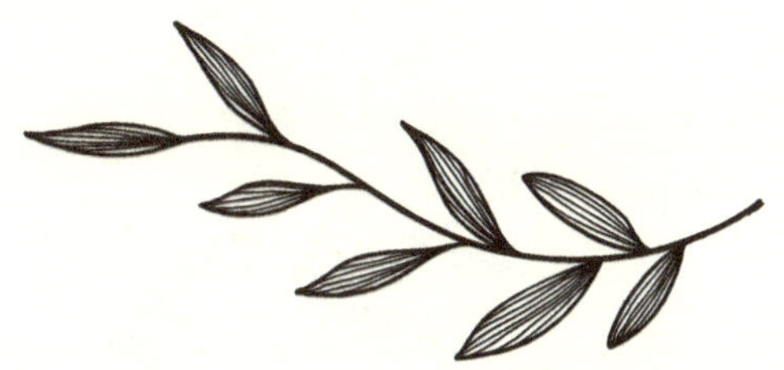

Echinacea Tincture

Ingredients: Echinacea root (Echinacea purpurea), alcohol (vodka or grain alcohol).

Process: Fresh or dried echinacea root is soaked in alcohol for 4–6 weeks in a sealed jar, shaken daily. Alcohol extracts the active compounds, such as polysaccharides and alkylamides, which stimulate the immune system.

Uses: This tincture is widely used for boosting the immune system, particularly at the onset of colds, flu, or infections. It helps the body fight off viruses and bacteria more effectively. Echinacea tincture can be taken daily during flu season as a preventive measure or at the first sign of illness.

Dosage: 30–40 drops (about 1 dropper full) in water, taken 2–3 times a day.

Valerian Root Tincture

Ingredients: Valerian root (Valeriana officinalis), alcohol (vodka or brandy).

Process: The root is chopped and soaked in alcohol for 4–6 weeks. The alcohol extracts valerian's active compounds, such as valerenic acid, which is known for its sedative and muscle-relaxing properties.

Uses: Valerian root tincture is a powerful remedy for insomnia, anxiety, and tension. It helps calm the nervous system, promoting deep, restful sleep, and can relieve muscle cramps or tension headaches.

Dosage: 30–40 drops in water or tea, taken 30 minutes before bed or during periods of high stress.

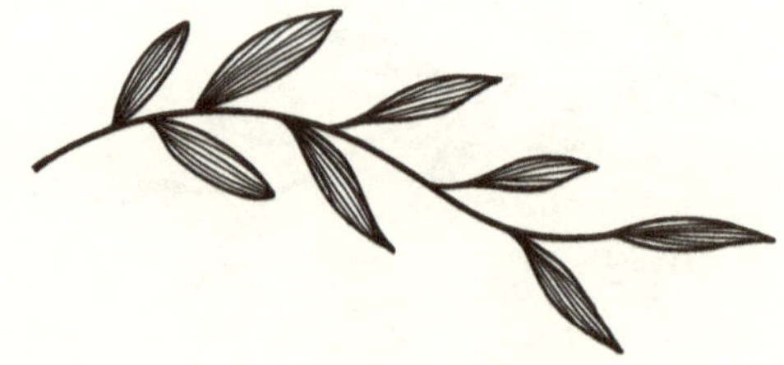

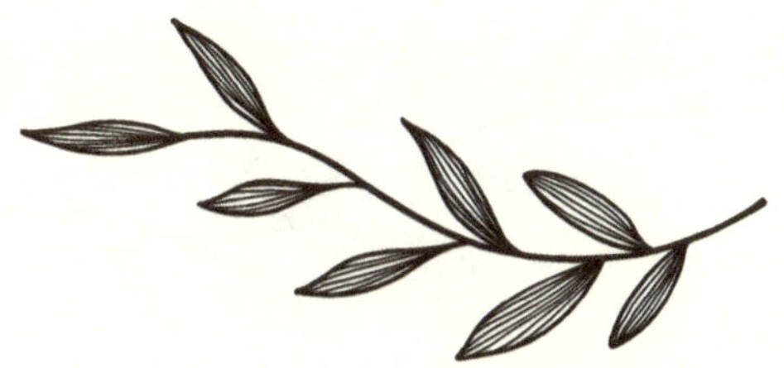

Turmeric Tincture

Ingredients: Fresh or dried turmeric root (Curcuma longa), alcohol (vodka or grain alcohol).

Process: Turmeric root is soaked in alcohol for 4–6 weeks, allowing the curcumin to be extracted. Curcumin is known for its anti-inflammatory, antioxidant, and pain-relieving properties.

Uses: Turmeric tincture is excellent for reducing inflammation in the body, making it beneficial for conditions like arthritis, joint pain, and digestive issues. It can also support liver detoxification and improve overall immunity.

Dosage: 15–30 drops in water or juice, 2–3 times a day, especially with food to enhance absorption.

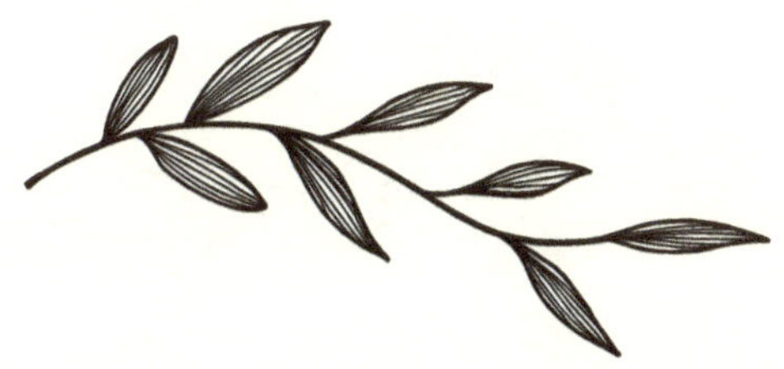

St. John's Wort Tincture

Ingredients: Fresh or dried St. John's Wort flowers (Hypericum perforatum), alcohol (vodka or brandy).

Process: Flowers are soaked in alcohol for 4–6 weeks. The active compounds, such as hypericin and hyperforin, are extracted, giving this tincture its mood-lifting properties.

Uses: St. John's Wort tincture is commonly used to alleviate mild to moderate depression, anxiety, and mood swings. It can also be applied topically for nerve pain or to help heal cuts and burns.

Dosage: 20–30 drops in water, taken 2–3 times a day for mood support. When using for depression, it may take a few weeks to notice full effects.

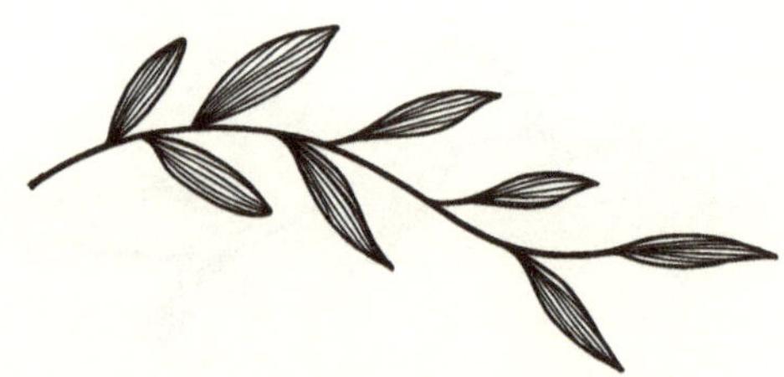

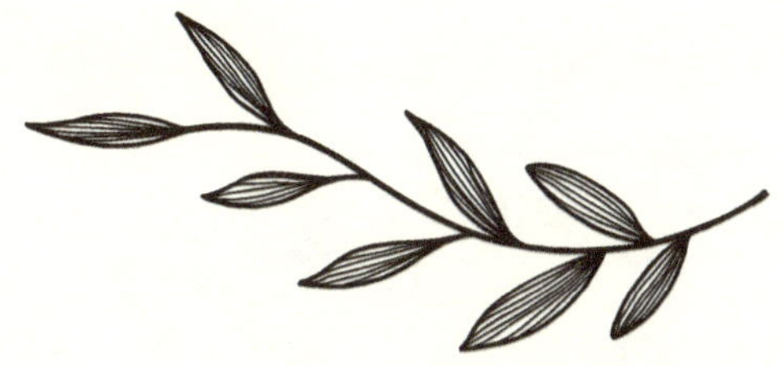

Ginger Tincture

Ingredients: Fresh ginger root (Zingiber officinale), alcohol (vodka or grain alcohol).

Process: Fresh ginger root is finely chopped and soaked in alcohol for 4–6 weeks. The alcohol extracts gingerol, the active compound responsible for ginger's anti-inflammatory and digestive benefits.

Uses: Ginger tincture is primarily used for nausea, motion sickness, and digestive issues. It's also a natural anti-inflammatory, making it useful for sore muscles and joint pain. It can boost circulation and help with cold symptoms.

Dosage: 20–30 drops in water or tea before meals to aid digestion, or at the first sign of nausea.

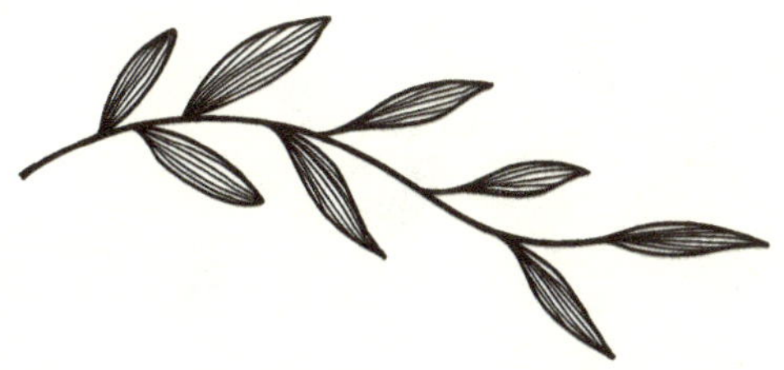

Ashwagandha Tincture

Ingredients: Dried ashwagandha root (Withania somnifera), alcohol (vodka or grain alcohol).

Process: The root is soaked in alcohol for 4–6 weeks, extracting withanolides, the compounds that give ashwagandha its adaptogenic properties.

Uses: Ashwagandha tincture is excellent for stress relief and balancing the body's response to anxiety. It helps improve sleep, enhance energy, and supports the adrenal system, making it useful for those experiencing burnout or chronic stress.

Dosage: 30–40 drops in water or juice, taken 1–2 times a day for overall stress management.

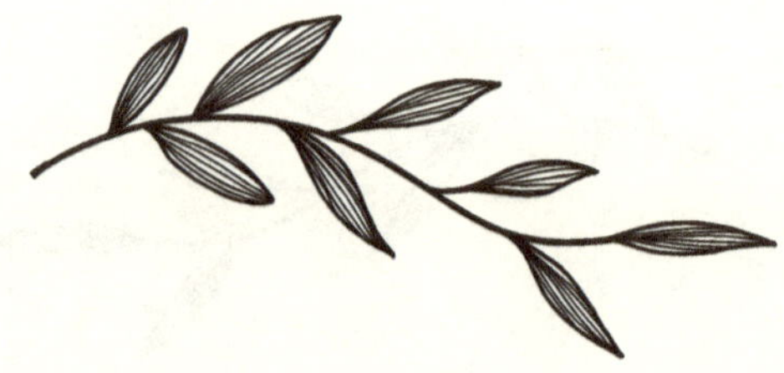

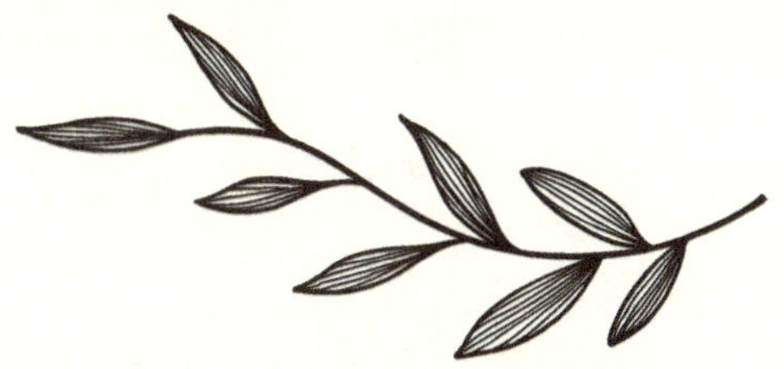

Milk Thistle Tincture

Ingredients: Milk thistle seeds (Silybum marianum), alcohol (vodka or grain alcohol).

Process: Milk thistle seeds are soaked in alcohol for 4–6 weeks, allowing silymarin, the active compound, to be extracted. Silymarin is known for its liver-protecting properties.

Uses: Milk thistle tincture is a powerful liver tonic, supporting detoxification and regeneration of liver cells. It is often used to treat liver conditions, cleanse the body after alcohol consumption, or during detox protocols.

Dosage: 20–30 drops in water or juice, 1–2 times a day for liver support.

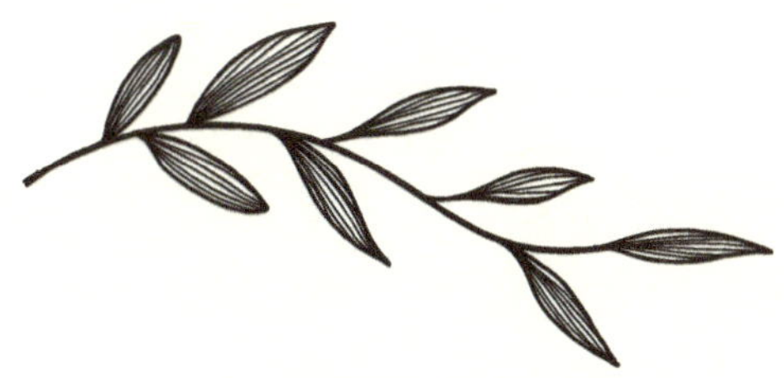

Tincture Date: ____________

Tincture Date: ___________

Tincture Date: ______________

Tincture Date: ______________

Tincture

Date: ______________

Tincture Date: ________________

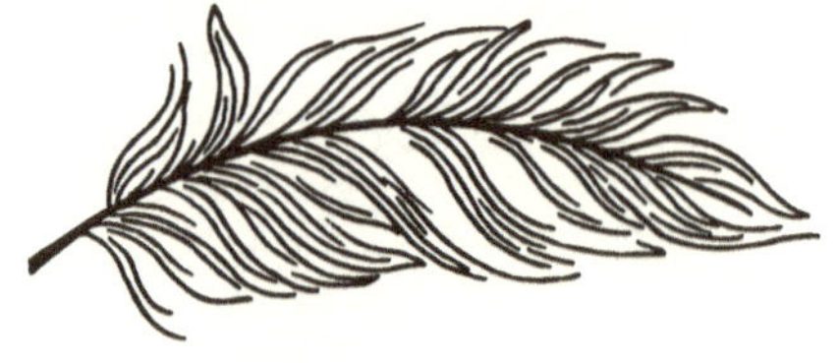

These tinctures are potent herbal extracts, each offering unique benefits. They should be used mindfully, and if you're new to herbal medicine, consult a healthcare provider before starting. Proper dosage and moderate use are key to gaining the most benefit without overwhelming the body.

Your Body is your temple
Take care of that sacred temple
Love and Peace

www.ingramcontent.com/pod-product-compliance
Lightning Source LLC
Chambersburg PA
CBHW051300250726
48656CB00004B/1402

9798300103453